SUKHAYU

The Ayurveda Way to a Healthy Life

DR. RAJMOHAN
B.A.M.S, M.D (Ayu)

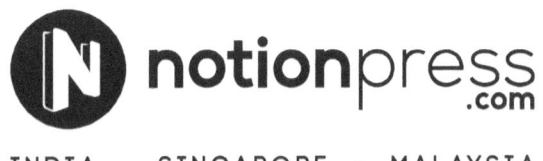

INDIA • SINGAPORE • MALAYSIA

Notion Press

Old No. 38, New No. 6
McNichols Road, Chetpet
Chennai - 600 031

First Published by Notion Press 2018
Copyright © Dr. Rajmohan 2018
All Rights Reserved.

ISBN 978-1-64249-400-6

This book has been published with all reasonable efforts taken to make the material error-free after the consent of the author. No part of this book shall be used, reproduced in any manner whatsoever without written permission from the author, except in the case of brief quotations embodied in critical articles and reviews.

The Author of this book is solely responsible and liable for its content including but not limited to the views, representations, descriptions, statements, information, opinions and references ["Content"]. The Content of this book shall not constitute or be construed or deemed to reflect the opinion or expression of the Publisher or Editor. Neither the Publisher nor Editor endorse or approve the Content of this book or guarantee the reliability, accuracy or completeness of the Content published herein and do not make any representations or warranties of any kind, express or implied, including but not limited to the implied warranties of merchantability, fitness for a particular purpose. The Publisher and Editor shall not be liable whatsoever for any errors, omissions, whether such errors or omissions result from negligence, accident, or any other cause or claims for loss or damages of any kind, including without limitation, indirect or consequential loss or damage arising out of use, inability to use, or about the reliability, accuracy or sufficiency of the information contained in this book.

WELCOME

Welcome to the World of Ayurveda.

The Ayurveda Way to a Healthy Life

"The way you think, the way you behave, the way you eat, can influence your life by 30 to 50 years is well known fact.

And to make it simple we can put it this way, Three F's are the reason for most of our health problems.

Fast Food, Fast Life, Fast Medicine are the reasons for the drop down in health.

Fast food: Junk, Oily, frozen, baked forms of food

Fast life: stress, no sleep, work-work-work

Fast medicine: due to lack of time and patience, people choose medicine, which gives quick relief, but in turn damages the body systems.

During the course of my clinical journey, I have witnessed all the sufferings of people, where people are still not aware about the cause of their problems.

The book do not discuss in depth about the different concepts of Ayurveda, as it may create confusions in the mind of readers since they are beginners.

Throughout the book I have described Ayurveda in the most practical way.

Wishing you a Happy Reading………

CONTENTS

Foreword — *vii*
Foreword — *ix*
Acknowledgments — *xi*

1. INTRODUCTION TO AYURVEDA — 1
2. BASIC CONCEPTS OF AYURVEDA — 11
3. THREE QUALITIES OF MIND — 27
4. FIVE ELEMENTS — 33
5. SEVEN TISSUES — 37
6. WASTE PRODUCTS OF THE BODY — 51
7. AGNI — 57
8. THREE PILLARS OF LIFE — 65
9. DAILY REGIMEN — 101
10. SEASONAL REGIMEN — 117
11. CLASSIFICATION OF TREATMENT ACCORDING TO AYURVEDA — 127
12. DETOXIFICATION THERAPIES — 131
13. EXTERNAL TREATMENTS IN AYURVEDA — 143
14. OLD AGE RELATED DISEASES — 151
15. MIDDLE AGE REALTED DISEASES — 161
16. YOUNG AGE RELATED DISEASES — 179
17. COMPLETE HEALTH CARE — 185

18.	CONCEPTS OF FOOD	241
19.	FRESH JUICES	249
20.	MEDICINAL JUICES	255
21.	MILK AND MILK PRODUCTS	259
22.	SOUPS	265
23.	TEA	273
24.	SALADS	279
25.	SANDWICH	285
26.	SAUCE	289
27.	SPECIAL LIGHT FOOD	295
28.	PANCAKE	303
29.	RICE DISHES	315
30.	DESSERTS	325
31.	SWEET PUDDINGS	335
32.	SWEET DRINKS	345
33.	NON VEGETARIAN DISHES	351
34.	AYURVEDA HOME REMEDIES	365

Dear Readers	*381*
Achievements	*383*

FOREWORD

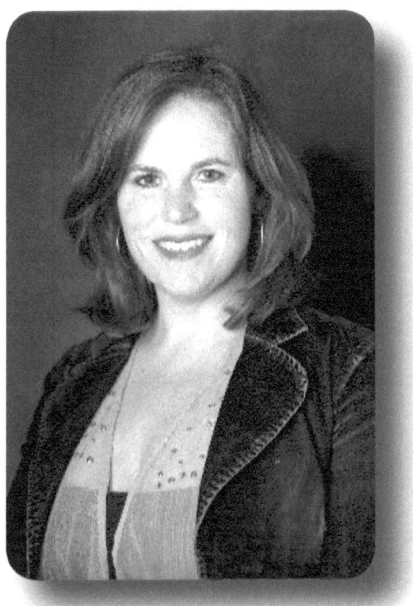

I am grateful that I have met Dr. Rajmohan at an Ayurvedic workshop in The Netherlands in 2017.

We've been friends since then.

At this workshop he shared his knowledge and spoke with passion about his profession.

Dr. Rajmohan gave extensive practical information.

He works very hard to support people in a conscious and healthy living and to bring this standard in Ayurvedic.

I am therefore very proud that he has written this book. His work will benefit the common people who do not know anything about Ayurveda.

I congratulate him and am proud to write the foreword for this book.

By reading this book, the common people can practice Ayurveda in their daily live and prevent them from diseases.

'It will change your life to a much more healthier and happier life.'

I wish Dr. Rajmohan all the best and a great success.

Kind regards,

Tessa van Dongen, Practice Gele Ster

Bachelor in Pedagogical-Social work and developer of Harmoni3 R

(Body-, Heart- and Mindfulness Training, Coaching and Education)

FOREWORD

I am blessed to be a mentor and guide to Dr. Rajmohan for the past 15 years.

He was found to be dedicated, hardworking under his training period under me, even during his bachelor degree days to mention.

I am happy and proud that he is writing a book in Ayurveda for the common people.

He has done lot of intensive reading, scientific interpretations and updates to reach the book practical and simple.

The book has explained the different concepts of Ayurveda with practical utility. He has tried to highlight the present day health issues and it's management through Ayurveda.

I am sure the book will surely help the common people to lead healthy life through this book.

I am proud to write the forward for his book.

I pray God to give blessings, prosperity, success, happiness and health to him.

– Dr. C.B. Vipinachandran Nair B.A.M
Changethu Bhaskaran Nair Memorial Hospital,
Thazhevettipuram,
Pathanamthitta (Dist), Kerala,
India – 689 645

ACKNOWLEDGMENTS

I would like to thank God for giving me this idea, determination, patience and making the book a reality.

My parents – for the constant support, encouragement and making me stand where am today.

My wife – for the constant support, igniting the fire and energy in me, healthy discussions and dedication throughout the process of the book and making it possible.

My brother- for the cooperation, support.

My father in law, mother in law – for the moral support, encouragement.

Mr. Noushadh (Silverhost), Mr. Mahesh Anaparthae – for providing the photos for the book.(Photo courtesy)

Dr. Vipin Chandran, Dr. L. Mahadevan – for the guidance, inspiration.

Mr. Kurup, Mr. Gireesh Menon: for the guidance,support behind the book.

Mr. Shameer Babu, Dr. Venu Sasikumar- for the support

Ms. Tessa Van Dongen – for writing the forward and constant support.

Mr. Frans Veltman, Ms. Jacqueline Hopstaken – for the constant support,understanding, encouragment.

Mr. Baby Mathew, Mr. Subash. C. Bose of Somatheeram Ayurveda village Hospital and Research Centre: for giving the idea, inspiration behind the book.

Mr. K.K. Krishnan, Mr. T.N. Raja: for their guidance and support.

Notion Press Team, Chennai: for valuable suggestions, guidance and publishing my book.

I thank all the staff of SDM College of Ayurveda, Udupi; Ayurveda community, my relatives, my friends for directly or indirectly be the cause of the book.

INTRODUCTION TO AYURVEDA

- ESSENCE OF THE BOOK   3
- AIM   3
- WHAT IS AYURVEDA? HOW DIFFERENT IS IT FROM OTHER SYSTEMS OF MEDICINE? IS AYURVEDA ONLY A TRADITIONAL FORM OF MEDICINE?   4
- AYURVEDIC TREATMENT PRINCIPLES   7
- ADJUVENTS   8
- OBJECTIVES OF AYURVEDA   9
- ORIGIN OF AYURVEDA   9
- EIGHT BRANCHES OF AYURVEDA   10

INTRODUCTION TO AYURVEDA

ESSENCE OF THE BOOK

- The book mainly focuses on how to understand Ayurveda in the simplest way and how to utilize Ayurveda in day to day life.
- The book contains description of the basic concepts of Ayurveda, the different stages of life like childhood, adolescence, old age and managing common diseases in the respective stages of life.
- The concepts like way of taking food, sleeping patterns, lifestyle management are also beautifully explained.
- The interesting and the most informative part in the book are the various healthy Food recipes.
- The language used in the book is simple, so it is easy to understand and interpret the given matter.

AIM

- The main Aim of the book is to reach out to the common people with the knowledge of Ayurveda, so that one can practice Ayurveda in their daily routine.
- The book aims to explain the scientific and logical reasoning behind the basic concepts of Ayurveda.

- The Book mainly aims to reach out to the common people who are unaware or partially aware about Ayurveda.

WHAT IS AYURVEDA? HOW DIFFERENT IS IT FROM OTHER SYSTEMS OF MEDICINE? IS AYURVEDA ONLY A TRADITIONAL FORM OF MEDICINE?

- A little bit of a deeper information of Ayurveda will erase all the questions.
- Ayurveda is the science of life, way of life, way to get closer to the nature and lead a qualitative and quantitative life.
- The text used in Ayurveda is mainly explained in the Sanskrit language with a lot of value and broader meaning.
- The text cannot be exactly correlated to the modern and scientific explanations, but for easy understanding we will try to make it simple.
- Ayurveda for an easy understanding is made up of two words namely *Ayu* and *Veda*.
- *Ayu* means life, whereas *Veda* means science.
- Thus Ayurveda means the science of life.
- It also tells about wholesomeness and unwholesomeness which brings happiness and sorrow to the body and mind.
- Ayurveda unlike other sciences mainly focuses on seizing the disease at the root cause rather than focusing on symptomatic treatment.
- It relieves symptoms as well as it arrests the further progression of the disease.
- Ayurveda stands out to be unique as it is a curative as well as preventive form of medicine.

Ayurveda Pharmaceutical Preparation

- Ayurveda medicines are mainly herbal and few are mineral based.
- When the medicines are processed properly and taken in the right dose, it can never have any side effects on the body.
- The plant as a whole or one main part is used in the preparation of Ayurveda medicines.
- There are various steps for collection, cleaning the herbs and different equipment like mortar and pestle, grinding machine, pulverizer, etc. which are used for making the medicines.

Different Forms of Ayurvedic Medicines

	Main forms of Ayurveda medicine	
English names	**Ayurveda terms**	**Examples**
Juice extract	*Swarasa*	Ginger juice, tulasi juice, aloe vera juice
Paste	*Kalka*	Neem paste, garlic paste
Decoction	*Kwatha*	Dashamoola kwatha, Rasnadi kwatha
Cold infusion	*Hima*	Dhanyaka hima, Sarivadi hima
Hot infusion	*Phanta*	Panchakola phanta
Powders	*Choorna*	Avipattikara choorna, Triphala choorna
Pills/Tablets	*Vati*	Dhanvantari vati, Chandraprabha vati
Semisolid jam	*Lehya*	Chyavanaprasha, Kushmanda rasayana
Fermented medicine	*Asava/Arishta*	Ushirasava, Draksharishta

Refer Fig 1.0

All these preparations are given in different conditions, in different time and different doses.

Mineral Medicines

- Minerals medicines are used less and in severe health conditions.
- There are few mineral medicines which are used in building up immunity and body strength.
- Minerals should be taken only after proper purification or it can cause toxicity to the body.
- According to Ayurveda minerals undergo many purification procedures, almost 7–10 times.
- There are many procedures which completely remove toxins and make it safe for use.
- Mineral medicines are prescribed in very small dose.
- Hence, it doesn't cause any toxicity or adverse effect and it will be safe for consumption.

Examples

§ Purified Gold

Used for increasing immunity and intelligence.

Eg: *Swarna bhasma*

§ Purified black bitumen used for building up immunity and vitality.

Eg: *Siddha makaradhwaja, Brihat vata chintamani rasa* with gold.

§ Purified Silver

To bulid up immunity, nerve tonic, health suppliment.

Eg: *Rajatha bhasma*

§ Purified Mercury

It is rejuvinative, strengthening and helps in wound healing, also has antimicrobial property.

Eg: *Arogyavardhini rasa*

§ Purified Sulphur

It is the best blood purifier, it is anti-bacterial. cures skin disorders, herpes, etc.

Eg: *Gandhaka rasayana, Gandhaka malahara*

§ Purified Iron

It is used as iron supplement in anemia, jaundice and body swelling.

Eg: *Punarnava mandoora, Dhatri loha*

§ Purified Coral

It is useful in treating respiratory disorders especially cold, cough, eye disorders and vaginal discharges.

Eg: *Pravala pishti*

§ Purified Oyster shell

It is the best calcium supplement and cures hyperacidity or colicky pain.

Eg: *Shankha bhasma*

AYURVEDIC TREATMENT PRINCIPLES

- Treatment in Ayurveda is not generalized but it is individualized.
- It is about finding
  1. The root cause of disease and avoiding the factors which triggers the disease.
  2. It is also about giving relief to the present health problems.
  3. It stops further progression of the disease.
- Ayurveda treatment depends upon the stage of the disease, patient's physical and mental strength.

- Ayurveda treatment also depends on other factors such as body constitution of the person, *dosha* imbalance etc.
- There are certain diseases which do not get relieved even after best treatments.
- By further understanding the depth of disease, the main cause is found to be the bad deeds of previous birth.
- After offerings to the God which is a ritual or other Ayurveda treatment modalities, the disease may relive.
- Ayurveda treatment becomes success not only by physician's efforts but also by the combined efforts of therapist, medicines and patient.
- The most important thing is patients mind strength, acceptance and belief in Ayurveda.
- In Ayurveda, medicines are not generalized, it is specific to condition.

Example

- In digestive problems, like low digestive fire, medicine is taken before or with the food.
- Similarly, in case of acidity, medicine is taken after food, if taken before food, it worsens the condition.
- In respiratory problems and diabetic conditions the medicine is taken frequently about 4–5 times a day.

ADJUVENTS

- Food when is dry, one feels like drinking water along with it and while we drink water we feel comfortable.
- Similarly medicines when taken simply will cause discomfort, whereas when it is taken with water it enters easily.

- Adjuvent (*Anupana*) is the drink which is taken along/after taking medicine.
- According to Ayurveda, medicine when taken with an after drink acts best on the body.
- Adjuvant helps medicine to act wonderfully on the body.
- The medicine gets absorbed very soon, hence action will be quick.

Example

- After taking pill, we drink warm water.
- Similarly, powder is mixed with honey and taken.

OBJECTIVES OF AYURVEDA

1. To maintain the health in healthy individual and treat the disease in diseased persons.
2. To attain *Dharma* (duty/virtue), *Artha* (wealth), *Kama* (desire), *Moksha* (salvation/liberation).
   - Ayurveda not only concentrates on the diseased condition, but also mainly focuses on maintaining health.
   - Maintenance of health being its prime motto by various factors which will be discussed in coming contexts.

ORIGIN OF AYURVEDA

- Ayurveda is said to be existed back in around 5000 B.C.
- Lord *Dhanwantari* is said to be the God of Ayurveda.

- Ayurveda originated in the Prehistoric times and some of the concepts existed from the time of Indus Valley civilization.
- Ayurveda developed significantly during the Vedic period and it is a discipline of *Upaveda*.
- The origin of Ayurveda is found in *Atharvaveda*.
- *Charaka Samhita*, *Susruta Samhita* and *Astanga Hridaya* are the main texts of Ayurveda.

EIGHT BRANCHES OF AYURVEDA

The eight branches of Ayurveda are
- *Kaya* (General medicine)
- *Bala* (Pediatrics)
- *Graha* (Psychology)
- *Urdhwanga* (Diseases of Ear, Nose, Throat)
- *Shalya* (Surgery)
- *Damshtra* (Toxicology)
- *Jara* (Geriatrics)
- *Vrusha* (Aphrodisiac)

BASIC CONCEPTS OF AYURVEDA

- THREE *DOSHA* (HUMOR) 13
- DESCRIPTION OF EACH *DOSHA* 14
- NOTE 25

BASIC CONCEPTS OF AYURVEDA

THREE *DOSHA* (HUMOR)

1. *VATA*
2. *PITHA*
3. *KAPHA*

- *Dosha* is humor in the body which maintains the body when it is in equilibrium and destroys the body when it is imbalanced.
- The three *doshas* mainly are *Vata, Pitha* and *Kapha*.

Body constitution *(Prakruthi)*

- Body constitution is a permanent constitution of a person.
- Body constitution is present or inherited in individual from birth by the combination of maternal and paternal factors.
- When there is disequilibrium in the body it is called *Vikruthi* (*doshas* in pathological state).

Factors that decide *Prakruthi* (Body constitution) of a person are

- *Shukra* (semen) from male and *Arthava* (ovum) from female.
- The state during the conception produces unique features in an individual (conceived product).

- There will be one in dominance as depending upon the *Shukra* (sperm), *Arthava* (ovum), pregnant lady's diet, activities, condition of uterus, and ovulation period.
- Thus a mother and father should follow healthy food, way of behavior and lifestyle when planning for a child.

DESCRIPTION OF EACH *DOSHA*

VATA

The qualities similar to that of air:
- Dry
- Light
- Cool
- Rough
- Subtle (property to penetrate through smallest possible space)
- Mobile

Function
- *Vata* means air. The air has movement; same way is the *Vata dosha* functions like different movements of the body.
- Smell sensation is another function of *Vata* dosha.
- *Vata dosha* can be compared to the Central Nervous system.
- *Vata dosha* normal function is that it is a controlling force/motivating force of life.
- *Vata dosha* is responsible for governing various voluntary and involuntary activities of body and speech.
- *Vata* controls and motivates the functions of the mind.

- It initiates the sense organs to perceive its respective senses.
- It maintains the respective position of tissues in the body, dries up the body.
- *Vata* is the reason for excitement or enthusiasm.
- *Vata* also governs functions like enthusiasm, expiration, inspiration, activities, initiates/regulates the natural urges.

Characteristics of person with dominant *Vata dosha*

- A person of *Vata dosha* typically will have lean body.
- The person of this *dosha* will have rough and dry skin/hair/nails, brownish hair and skin.

Characteristic: Even if the person eats more he doesn't tend to gain more weight.

Mental status

- *Vata* person's main character is instability of mind.
- His/her mind keeps on wandering like bird.
- Such persons will have lack of concentration, hyperactive in mind.
- Way of dealing: person wants the things to be done very soon.
- Person takes quick initiation in work, but would make it incomplete or quit in the half way.
- A person possessing this nature will have lack of confidence, lack of motivation, lack of self-esteem.
- So these people are more prone to Depression, Anxiety and sleep disorders.
- The person grasps very soon and same way forgets it fast.
- The digestive capacity will be irregular, will have constipated or hard stools.

- Irregularity in sleep, bowel, digestion, and thinking is the main feature of *Vata dosha*.
- The person's voice will be harsh or rough, with high pitch.
- Joint movements and walking will be irregular, (/very fast).
- The joint emits sound or roughness while performing day to day activities.
- The *Vata* can be mainly correlated to Central Nervous system of body.

Locations of *Vata dosha* in body

- The locations of *Vata* are Intestine, hips, lower limbs, sense organ of hearing (ear), and sense organ of touch (skin).
- Intestine forms the most important location of *Vata*.

PITHA

The qualities of *Pitha dosha* are similar to that of the fire element.

- Unctuous
- Sharp
- Hot
- Light
- Clear
- Liquid

Function

- The word *Pitha* reminds of heat.
- *Pitha* is the one responsible for digestion, its heat and warm quality is responsible for body temperature.
- *Pitha* regulates intelligence, consciousness, grasping power.

- *Pitha* is also responsible for vision, hunger, thirst, taste, and lustre, retention of memory, perception, intellect and strength.

Characteristics of person with predominant *Pitha dosha*

- A person with predominance of *Pitha* is moderately built.
- The body temperature is very warm, so the person sweats heavily.
- Hence these persons will have characteristic bad body smell.
- Skin is moderately oily and sweaty.
- The person tends to have a strong appetite with a strong digestive power.
- This person drinks more water as well as gets hungry soon.
- The person having *Pitha dosha* doesn't tend to gain much weight.
- These persons are more prone to skin problems like pimples, skin rashes in underarm, in between thighs etc.

Mental status

- Person with *Pitha dosha* has stable mind.
- These person are stubborn, short tempered, have good concentration power and aggressive.

Way of dealing

- *Pitha dosha* person are very quick in decisions making, very punctual and systematic.
- This person always talk to the point, has leadership qualities.
- This person gets aggressive thoughts, and are revengeful.
- *Pitha dosha* person grasps moderately fast and can retain for some time.
- Digestive capacity: will be very strong with much frequency in stools or increased bowel movements.
- Person with *Pitha dosha* will have sharp, high pitched and louder voice.

- Joint movements being stable, faster yet steady, warm joints.
- *Pitha* can be mainly correlated to Endocrine system and Digestive system.
- *Pitha* persons by their short temperedness and aggressiveness are more prone to high blood pressure, Stress, Insomnia.
- And by their hot body temperature, they are prone to skin problems, Acidity.

Locations of *Pitha dosha* in body

- The locations of *Pitha* dosha are the umbilical region, stomach, sweat, plasma, serum, lymphatic, blood, vision, touch. The main location of *Pitha* is umbilicus.

KAPHA

The qualities of *Kapha dosha* are similar to that of earth element.

- Unctuous
- Cool
- Heavy
- Slow
- Fine
- Sticky
- Stable

Function

- The word *Kapha* symbolizes heaviness.
- *Kapha* dosha is a potential source of power and strength.
- *Kapha* is responsible for the bulky structure of body.

Characteristics of person with predominant *Kapha dosha*

- Person with *Kapha dosha* are well built.
- The body temperature of person with *Kapha* is cold and has smooth skin.
- Person has moderate appetite, digestion power is poor.
- Person have a comparatively clear and glowing skin.
- The skin is often prone to itching with watery discharge.

Mental status

- *Kapha dosha* person will be stable minded and calm.
- *Kapha dosha* person will be having good temperament and patience.
- They have very good concentration power with excellent retaining capacity.
- Way of dealing: *Kapha dosha* person are cool headed, slow to initiate activities and work.
- These person if initiated, finishes work in perfect manner.
- Digestive capacity: will be moderate with good absorption capacity.
- *Kapha dosha* person tend to gain weight more easily.
- Their voice will be heavier, low pitched and smooth.
- Their movements are slow and steady.
- *Kapha dosha* can be mainly correlated to Muscular, Adipose tissue system.

Locations of *Kapha dosha* in body

- The main locations of *Kapha dosha* are chest, neck, head, pancreas, joints, stomach, and plasma.
- The other locations are adipose tissue, nose, and tongue.
- *Kapha dosha* main location being the chest region.

Characteristics	VATA	PITHA	KAPHA
Skin and complexion	Dry and scaly Dull, darkish, complexion	Oily and smooth Moles, pigments Yellowish fair	Oily and soft Clear skin Fair color
Built	Thin and hyposthenic	Moderate and normosthenic	Compact body and strong and hypersthenic
Gait	Fast-unsteady or irregular	Fast yet steady	Steady and stern
Joints	Crepitating and cold on touch	Stern and warm on touch	Stern and cold in touch
Activities	Quick initiation Quick progress Hyperactive	Quick initiation Moderate progress Lively or active	Slow initiation Slow progress Sedentary or lazy
Features			
• Forehead	Broad and wide Dry, smoke color	Broad or medium Watery, reddish color	Narrow, covered with hairs Shiny, whitish colored
• Eyes	Shape round	Small sharp eyes	Big prominent eyes
• Lips	Dry, rough, cracked	Soft, Reddish colour	Soft, wet lips
• Face cut	Thin and long face	Moderately long and small face	Round and broad face
• Voice	Hoarse, cracked voice	Sharp, loud voice	Heavy, sweet voice
• Height	Tall	Medium	Short
Strength	Very less	Moderate	Very good
Sexual life	Reduced libido Less children	Reduced libido Will have less children	Increased libido Will have many children
Food intake & Digestion	Frequent food intake, yet less quantity Weak digestion	Large quantity of food intake Very good digestion	Moderate quantity of food intake Moderately good digestion
Bowel habits	Constipated, once in 2–3 days	Soft bowel, 2–3 times a day	Soft bowel, Once a day
Sleep	Sleeps very less Sleeps late at night and wakes up late in morning	Sleeps moderate Sleeps early and wakes up early	Sleeps almost all the time Sleeps early and wakes up late
Intellect and memory	Poor intellect Least memory power	Excellent intellect Moderate memory power	Excellent intellect Great memory power

Characteristics	VATA	PITHA	KAPHA
Decision making	Fluctuating, can't reach to conclusion	Takes decision quickly May retain or change (but wise)	Takes decision slowly yet tries to retain it for long
Life span	Short	Medium	Long

Food suitable for person having predominant *Vata dosha*

- *Vata dosha* persons will have a dry body, digestion being irregular.
- People suffer from slight to fully constipated bowels.
- Food with qualities like hot, sharp, soft, unctuous (fat rich), heavy, and sweet, sour, salty are suitable to maintain *Vata dosha*.
- Food like dry, light, cold, hard qualities are to be avoided as it worsens the digestive power and health of the person.
- Forms of food like soups, porridge, more fiber rich food, or laxative food are necessary.

Diet for *Vata dosha*			
Cereals	Brown rice		
	Basmati rice or long grain rice		
	Njavara rice (red type of rice)		
	Wheat		
Legumes	Black gram		
	Sesame seeds		
Vegetable	Carrot	Ash gourd	
	Cucumber	green beans	
	Tamarind		
Fruits	Grapes	Pomegranate	papaya
	Mango	Indian gooseberry	Banana
	Coconut	pineapple	apple
	Orange		

22 | Sukhayu

	Diet for *Vata dosha*		
Dairy products	Whole milk	butter	Cheese
	Cream	ghee	Cottage cheese
	Yogurt	Lassi (sweet curd)	
Oils	Coconut oil	Flaxseed oil	Sunflower oil
	Sesame oil	Lemon oil	Nutmeg butter
	Olive oil	Apricot oil	apple
Herbs	Fennel	Onion	
	Curry leaves	Ginger	
	Basil leaves	Garlic	
Spices	Asafetida	Clove	
	Turmeric	Cardamom	
	Clove	Cumin	
Meat	Pork	Swan	Rabbit
	Beef	Duck	
	Buffalo	Turkey	
Sea food	Sardine	Shark	Kingfish

Food suitable for person having predominant *Pitha dosha*

- *Pitha* persons will have a warm body, digestion extremely good.
- There will be increased frequency and soft bowels.
- Food with qualities like soft, sweet, bitter is suitable.
- Food like dry, light, hot, are to be avoided as it worsens the digestive power and health of the person.
- Forms of food like juices, cool temperature food are to be consumed.

	Diet for *Pitha dosha*
Cereals	Rice
	Wheat
	Barley
	Oats

	Diet for *Pitha dosha*		
Lentils	Green gram		
	Bean seed		
	Chick peas (Bengal gram)		
Vegetables	Ash gourd	Radish	
	Pumpkin	Bitter gourd	
	Long beans	Asparagus	
	Carrot	Spinach	
	Cucumber		
Fruits	Peaches	Melon	Kiwi
	Cherries	Pomegranate	Strawberry
	Grapes	Coconut	Watermelon
	Pears	Blueberry	
Dairy products	Milk of cow and buffalo		
	Butter		
	Ghee		
Herbs	Curry leaves	Celery	
	Mint leaves	Lettuce	
	Methi leaves (fenugreek)	Vetiver roots	
Seeds	Flaxseed	poppy seeds	
	Pumpkin seeds	almond	
Spices	Turmeric	Coriander	
	Saffron	cardamom	
Meat	Mutton	Pigeon	
	Rabbit	Turkey	
	Sheep	Partridges	
	Deer	Quail	
Sea food	King fish Sardine, Sea weed		

Food suitable for person having predominant *Kapha dosha*

- *Kapha* persons will have a low body temperature, digestion being very less.
- Food with qualities like hot, dry, bitter, astringent light is suitable.
- Forms of food like oily, heavy, sweet are to be avoided as it worsens the digestive power and health of the person.

\	Diet for *Kapha dosha*		
Cereals	Red rice		
	Oats		
	Millet		
	Barley		
Lentils	Green gram		
	Horse gram		
	Masoor dal		
Vegetables	Bitter gourd	Green beans	Broccoli
	Cauliflower	Radish	
	Tomato	Cabbage	
Fruits	Blueberry	Apple	
	Lemon	Apricot	
	Orange	Coccum fruit	
Dairy products	Fat free cow's milk or diluted		
	Goats milk		
	Camels milk		
Oils	Ghee processed with bitter herbs like neem, snake gourd		
	Coconut oil	Olive oil	
	Mustard oil	Sesame oil	
Herbs	Fenugreek leaves		
	Curry leaves		
	Mint leaves		
	Leaves of chilli plant		
	Leaves of spring onion		

	Diet for *Kapha dosha*	
Seeds	Fennel seeds	Walnuts
	Mustard leaves	Hazel nuts
	Sesame seeds	
	Pumpkins seeds	
Spices	Ginger	Cardamom
	Turmeric	Clove
	Cinnamon	Garlic
Meat	Camel	Duck meat
	Ostrich	Lean meat
	Chicken (without fat)	
Sea food	Oyster, shrimp, squid	

NOTE

- Humans are made of all this three *doshas*, as each does its own function in the body. But each individual have mainly two predominant *doshas*.
- This body constitution is known as ones *Prakruti* which is permanent.
- The approximate percentage of the two *doshas* is difficult to understand.
- In a diseased condition, any particular two *doshas* are imbalanced.

THREE QUALITIES OF MIND

- POSITIVE MIND   29
- AGGRESSIVE MIND   30
- DULL MIND   31

THREE QUALITIES OF MIND

§ Positive mind (*Satvik*)

§ Aggressive mind (*Rajasik*)

§ Dull mind (*Tamasik*)
- The three qualities are present in the mind.
- It would be impossible for the mental function to go on without any of these qualities.
- But each one in his mind will have difference or predominance of one quality over the other two qualities.

POSITIVE MIND

- Positive mind is the reason to be very pleasant, being happy.
- People having such a mind will be free from desires, free from enmity and all worldly negativities.
- Person with predominance of this quality of mind will be happy, knowledgeable, and aware of truth of life.
- Person will be free from desires which would ruin the mind.
- Stability of the mind is the main quality, which makes the person intelligent and having good patience.

- It is the reason for joy, enlightenment and being a motivating force to others.
- One should maintain this quality by indulging more into prayers, meditation and by avoiding spicy, oily, heavy food.

AGGRESSIVE MIND

- Aggressive mind is the most common quality of mind.
- In the present era if one analyzes properly, each individual is bound under stress.
- Every human has strong expectations from others.
- In work there is too much pressure on employees to reach high level of targets.
- A person works for more than 10 hours which causes exhaustion.
- At home there will be expectations from parents/wife/husband/children.
- Thus the person gets fully exhausted and he will have further stress.
- He/She have no rest in mind.
- His/her mind will be further under stress.
- Thus there will be more aggression in thinking, decision, interaction.
- Aggressive mind is the reason for being violent, furious, selfish, congested mindset.
- Such a mind will be having too much ambition, materialistic.
- Person with predominance of this quality will be filled with anger, emotionally very fluctuating or least stable.

- This person is self-centered, desire for having everything and more than required, with no peace of mind, far from truth of life.
- Person should get rid of such mindset by indulging more into meditation and yoga especially *Yoga Nidra*.
- They should also avoid spicy and non-vegetarian food and eat vegetarian food.

Refer Fig 1.1

DULL MIND

- Dull mind/lazy mind is the reason for being very dull, ignorant, attached, fearful, with full of negativity.
- Person with predominance of this quality will be having lot of lethargy to initiate activities or thinking.
- This person is always sad, having congested thoughts and always emotional.
- This kind of character leads to agony, Depression.
- The person of this nature will have lack of knowledge, lack of awareness.
- One should get rid of dull and negative thinking by practicing Meditation, spiritual activities like praying God.
- This person should eat food which would make mind active.
- Food like bitter, sour, spicy should be taken in moderate quantity.
- Avoid sweet, heavy, and oily food as it makes a person more dull and lazy.

Refer Fig 1.2

FIVE ELEMENTS

- EARTH   36
- WATER   36
- FIRE   36
- AIR   36
- SPACE   36

FIVE ELEMENTS

The whole universe is made of the 5 elements.

Humans, plants, animals are all comprised of the five elements but in variable proportion.

The five elements are **Earth, Water, Fire, Air or Wind, Space.**

- In Ayurveda, herbs are being mainly used for treatment.
- The herbs are grown in the nature and are mainly composed of the five elements.
- In Ayurveda the herbs are used to treat the diseases.
- If an individual observes clearly, there are similarities in composition of five elements and herbs.
- If there is no water, there is no life.
- Similarly if there is no fire there is no body temperature and so on.
- Human body is made of three energies, which is again composed of five elements.

§ *Vata dosha*: Air + Space

§ *Pitha dosha:* Fire + Air

§ *Kapha dosha*: Earth + Water

In Ayurveda the treatment materials adopted such as the herbs, oil, ghee etc. all are made of these five elements and thus on same strategy it is used.

Five elements in relation with sense organs and its aspects

Earth = nose (smell)

- Earth is heavy, intact, and solid which provides stability, strength to the body.
- E.g.: bone

Water = tongue (taste)

- Water is moist, sticky and one with flowing nature.
- Thus it cleanses the body and keeps the body hydrated or moist.
- E.g.: fluid in the body.

Fire = eye (vision)

- Fire is hot, sharp, intense quality which increases the digestive fire, maintaining body temperature and metabolism of the body.
- E.g.: metabolism like digestive fire, body temperature, complexion etc.

Air = skin (sensation)

- Air is dry, light, transparent, rough quality which is responsible for the different body movements.
- E.g.: movement of the matter like blood flow, secretions in the gland, contraction of muscles

Space = ear (hearing)

- Space is hollow, smooth, subtle quality which is responsible to maintain the space within the hollow body areas like artery, nerves etc.
- E.g.: body cavities like intestine, intercellular space.

If any of these five elements are affected, then we can balance the disturbance by substituting the same source from the nature.

SEVEN TISSUES

- PLASMA/LYMPH (*RASA*) 39
- BLOOD/CIRCULATION SYSTEM (*RAKTA*) 41
- MUSCULAR SYSTEM/LIGAMENTS/TENDON (*MAMSA*) 42
- FAT/ADIPOSE TISSUE (*MEDA*) 44
- BONE/HAVERSIAN SYSTEM (*ASTHI*) 46
- BONE MARROW TISSUE (*MAJJA*) 47
- SPERM/OVUM/MENSTRUAL CYCLE OR REPRODUCTIVE SYSTEM (*SHUKRA*) 48

SEVEN TISSUES

1. Plasma/Lymph
2. Blood
3. Muscle
4. Fat/adipose tissue
5. Bone
6. Bone marrow
7. Sperm/ovum

Seven tissues are basic built up of the body. They maintain the structure, function, composition of the body.

The seven tissues are lymph, blood, muscle, adipose tissue, bone, bone marrow and sperm/ovum.

PLASMA/LYMPH (*RASA*)

- Plasma is the first tissue in body, whose function is to satisfy the needs of body.
- When it functions normally the body is healthy and when it increases or decreases then body gets afflicted with diseases.
- This tissue has more water content and smoothness in it. Both should be balanced so as to keep this tissue normal.

Reason for abnormalities

Increased plasma

- The digestive fire within the body increases due to food intake such as fat rich, protein rich fried as well as baked.
- Foods also like excessive sweets, more of salt or pickles, salted mango, beetroot or other vegetables also increase this tissue.
- Intake of all these food gives rise to conditions such as increased salivation, lethargy, heaviness.
- Pale color in body, decrease in the body temperature (cold skin/hypothermia), loose joints/organs, dyspnea, cough, increased sleep are the other conditions.

Decreased plasma

- Intake of dry food like biscuits, bread, chilled food, chilled drinks or juices, stored or preserved food stuffs in the body leads to dryness or reduced moisture content in the body.
- This leads to dehydration, dryness in body, dizziness or giddiness, loss of body weight, weak or tired feeling, irritability towards sounds.

Measures to be taken when lymph tissue is increased

- Food which helps to remove excess water retention and which increases digestive fire are to be taken.
- Foods having sharp quality, light and moderate dry food substances such as rice porridge with pepper, cumin are to be taken.
- Herbs and spices which increase appetite like ginger, garlic are to be consumed.
- One should reduce salt, sweet consumption.

Measures to be taken when lymph tissue is decreased

- Food with increased liquid content like water, salt and sweet, juices, grapes and pomegranate, raisins, figs, apricot are to be taken.
- Food intake of chicken soup, mutton soup helps in fluid regain and increased moisture content.

BLOOD/CIRCULATION SYSTEM (*RAKTA*)

- Blood is the second tissue of the body which reminds us about red color.
- Blood influences at the level of body (as it flows from heart and reaches throughout the body including brain) and mind.
- This tissue is made up of mainly fire element.
- *Pitha dosha* is related to that of the blood.
- Blood provides liveliness in the body.

Reasons for abnormalities

Increased blood tissue

- When the heat in the form of *Pitha dosha* is increased in the body, it give rise to the following below.
- Liver disorders, Cellulitis, splenomegaly, Abscesses, skin diseases, inflammatory joint disorders, bleeding disorders, extra growth in abdominal organs.
- Bleeding gums, Jaundice, Hyper pigmentation of face, reduced digestive fire, altered consciousness, reddish discoloration of skin, eyes, urine are the other conditions.

Decreased blood tissue

- Decreased blood tissue causes coldness in the body, desire for eating sour and cold food substances.
- There will be laxity in the blood vessels, skin dryness and roughness, reduction urine, stools and sweat production.

Measures to be taken to reduce the vitiation in blood

- When *Pitha dosha* is increased in the blood, the food which pacifies the *Pitha dosha* in the blood are to be adopted.
- Food and drinks of sweet, bitter should be taken like milk, butter, ghee, water melon, pomegranate, grapes, raisins, carrot, and spinach.
- Berries, mint, coconut water, Indian gooseberry, cherries, fennel seeds or leaves, neem, bitter gourd are also to be taken.

Measures to be taken to increase the blood tissue

- Foods which increase the digestive fire and reduced *Pitha dosha* should be taken.
- Food which also enhances the blood circulation and count are to be eaten.
- Cereals, lentils, beans, horse gram, spinach, dried raisins, green leafy vegetables, nuts, meat like chicken, mutton are to be taken.
- Fish, adequate pepper, ginger and garlic, turmeric and tamarind, neem (increases blood count as well as purifies blood), beetroot, broccoli, turmeric, onion, Indian gooseberry, ash gourd, cow's urine should also be taken.

MUSCULAR SYSTEM/LIGAMENTS/TENDON (*MAMSA*)

- Muscle is the third tissue of the body.
- Muscle is mainly made up of earth and fire elements.

- Muscle forms the protective covering to the bones, joints, vessels etc. structures and other systems.

Reason for abnormalities

Increased muscle tissue

- The *Kapha dosha* when increased has direct effect on the digestive fire or metabolism.
- Thus it leads to reduced digestion and metabolism.
- Increased muscle tissue causes stiff and hypertrophied muscular structures in the body.
- Diseases affecting neck region like Goiter, Cervical lymphadenitis, Large Malignant or Benign tumor, lumps, Lymphoma, Obesity, Metabolic syndrome are caused.

Decreased muscle tissue

- Decreased muscle tissue leads to very thin or weak muscle formation resulting in Chronic fatigue syndrome, muscle wasting, and loss of fat over cheeks, buttocks regions.

Measures to reduce increased muscle tissue

- Food which is sharp and light like vegetables and seeds are preferred.
- The spicy taste food is best as it lights up the digestive fire and brings down the increased muscle tissue.
- E.g.: Ginger, pepper, cinnamon, Piper longum used. Ones should consume hot and spicy vegetable soup like radish.
- Physical exercise and yoga are excellent ways to reduce the excess muscle tissue.

Measures to increase depleted muscle tissue

- Muscle tissue is decreased due to decreased metabolism.
- Food substances having heavy, cool, unctuous qualities which increase muscle tissue as well as metabolism should be taken.
- E.g.: Diary products like milk, butter, ghee, cheese, and yogurt.
- Meat like red meat (beef, pork, mutton), chicken, fish, shrimps.
- Vegetables like ash gourd, underground tubers like potato, cassava, yams.
- Avocado, nuts and dry fruits like raisins, dates, peanuts, badam, pistachios, figs.
- Rice, different types of dal like toor dal, ragi.
- The food explained above should be consumed.
- Pranayama and yoga are to be practiced.

FAT/ADIPOSE TISSUE (*MEDA*)

- Fat tissue is the fourth tissue in the body which increases the bulk of the body.
- It is composed mainly of water and earth elements.
- Body fat is responsible for providing bulk (bulkiness) to the body.

Reason for abnormalities

Increased fat tissue

- The increased intake of food having heavier qualities leads to greater amount of body fat in the body.
- The tissue fire which is responsible for fat tissue metabolism will be reduced.

- The impaired tissue metabolism causes heaviness in the body resulting in minimal activities.
- Fatigue, Dyspnea even on slight exertion, sagging of buttocks, belly, chest region (breast) are common conditions.

Decreased fat tissue

- Reduced body fat, thin body structure, numbness over the hip region, Spleenomegaly, emaciation is the conditions caused when there is decreased fat tissue.

Measures that reduce excess fat tissue

- The *Kapha dosha* is increased here leading to increased body fat.
- Food substances having qualities like sharp, bitter and astringent tastes are recommended here.
- Eg: Cinnamon, turmeric, kokum (Garcinia indica), juice of vegetables like ash gourd, bitter gourd, bottle gourd, green tea, pepper, ginger water.
- Water mixed with honey, fenugreek seeds, blue berries, broccoli, spinach, Olive oil, flax seed, and walnut are also beneficial here.
- *Triphala* is widely used in Ayurveda to reduce excess weight.
- Exercises like walking, cycling, *and Yoga* should be done.

Measures that increase body fat tissue

- Depletion of the fat tissues is seen here.
- Food substances having qualities like unctuous, sweet, strengthening.
- Grains like Rice, Wheat, Ragi, *Ashwagandha* (Withania somnifera), milk especially fat rich, cholustrum, buffalo milk, milk products, egg, cheese, yogurt.
- Reduced body exercise, more hours of sleep is beneficial to gain weight.

BONE/HAVERSIAN SYSTEM (*ASTHI*)

- Bone is fifth tissue in the body.
- Bone supports the body like that of pillar providing stability to the body.
- It is composed of earth and space elements.

Reason for abnormalities

Increased bone formation

- The digestive fire nourishing the bone tissue is affected, due to increase in *Kapha dosha*.
- Increased bone formation leads to denser and thicker bones.
- Extra teeth formation, Extra calcification/ossification like Calcaneal spur, Ankylosing spondylitis are the conditions.

Decreased *Asthi*

- The hot and sharp qualities of *Pitha dosha* is aggravated leading to decreased bone formation.
- Bone becomes narrower and weaker.
- The dry quality of *Vata* dosha increases, which is another factor leading to improper bone formation.
- The health conditions arising are shooting pain or stabbing pain in bone, falling of teeth, hairs, nails, weak bones; fractures, degenerative changes in younger age.

Measures that reduce excess bone tissue

- When there is an increase of *Kapha dosha* it leads to increased bone formation.
- Foods having qualities like light, sharp, hot and dry properties are to be opted in this condition.

- Foods having bitter taste like amaranth, spinach, bitter gourd, snake gourd are preferred here.
- Foods having pungent or spicy taste like pepper, cinnamon, asafetida, and other spices are beneficial here.

Measures that increase the decreased bone tissue

- A diet with more cooling properties are to be chosen like milk, butter, ghee, cheese, or dairy products.
- Wheat, rice, beans.
- Fat rich, sweet tasting, nutritious foods are to be taken
- One should consume milk and milk products, soya bean, okra, broccoli, wheat, spinach, eggs.
- Fishes like sardines, pink salmon; shrimp, egg shell and oyster shell powder (as a result of burnt shell) are to be taken.
- Meat like mutton especially in the form of soup, nuts like almond, cashew are also beneficial.

BONE MARROW TISSUE (*MAJJA*)

- Bone marrow is the sixth tissue of body, made up of earth and space element.
- Bone marrow fills the hollow structure in the bone.

Reason for abnormalities

Increased bone marrow tissue

- The increased intake of food having heavier qualities leads to increased bone marrow tissue.
- Increased bone marrow tissue causes heaviness in the eyes and parts of body, reddish brown eruptions over the joint.

Decreased bone marrow tissue

- The digestive fire responsible for the formation of bone marrow tissue is decreased leading to decreased bone marrow tissue.
- Decreased bone marrow tissue causes reduced bone density conditions like Osteoporosis, Osteomyelitis, Multiple sclerosis, diminished vision.

Measures that balances the increased bone marrow

- Foods having sweet taste, fat rich having heavier quality are to be taken.
- Foods like bitter and pungent are also to be used.
- Green leafy vegetables, juices of spinach, bitter gourd and fasting are most beneficial, with lots of fluid intake.
- Meat soups of mutton, meat of chicken are to be taken.

Measures taken to increase the reduced bone marrow tissue

- Food which is sweet, cooling, nourishing are to be taken in the diet.
- Foods like ghee, butter, milk, vegetables with bitter taste like amaranth leaves, bitter gourd, snake gourd, curry leaves, spinach, Brussels, fenugreek leaves are to be used in the diet.
- Nuts, figs and meat, fishes, eggs, food rich in vitamin B12 are also to be taken in the diet.

SPERM/OVUM/MENSTRUAL CYCLE OR REPRODUCTIVE SYSTEM (*SHUKRA*)

- Sperm/ovum is the seventh and last tissue of the body.
- This particular tissue is said to be the essence of all the six tissues, responsible for reproduction.

- It is basically predominant of earth and water elements.
- It can be correlated to male and female reproductive system.

Reason for abnormalities

- The factors like colour, volume, count, motility varies according to disturbance of *doshas* responsible.
- In males, **color of sperm indicates** the predominance of *dosha* accordingly like
    1. If the color is grey, it is predominant of *Vata dosha*,
    2. Yellowish color is predominant of *Pitha dosha*,
    3. Pale white color is predominant of *Kapha dosha*.

Based on volume of sperm,

- Reduced volume of sperm: *Vata dosha* predominant
- Medium volume of sperm: *Pitha dosha* predominant
- Large volume of sperm: *Kapha dosha* predominant

Based on count of sperm and motility (microscopic examination)

- Low count and motility of the sperm is caused by *Vata* dosha or *Pitha dosha*.
- Normal count and low motility of sperm is maintained by *Kapha dosha*.

In women,

- Ovum is called as *Arthava* or *Raja*.
- On examination of menstruation,
- If there is menstrual irregularity or Amenorrhea or Dysmenorrhea then *Vata dosha* is likely to be vitiated.
- If the menstrual flow is more, then *Pitha dosha* is vitiated.

- If menstrual flow is associated with clots or mucosal discharge then it is vitiated by *Kapha dosha.*

Measures that maintains *Shukra*

- When the reproductive tissues are vitiated by *Vata dosha* or Pitha *dosha*, a proper diet that ensures the nourishment and quantity are to be consumed.
- Food with sweet taste, fat rich like milk, ghee, butter, yogurt with sweetening agent mixed, nut are most beneficial.
- Banana, Indian gooseberry, pomegranate, tomatoes, pumpkin, avocado, black gram, walnuts, milk, yogurt, egg, meat of mutton, chicken, pork, beef, fish are the best food.
- Best aphrodisiac (sexual capacity promoter) are Herbs like *Ashwagandha.*

WASTE PRODUCTS OF THE BODY

- WASTE PRODUCTS (THREE *MALA*)   53
- SWEAT (*SWEDA*)   53
- URINE (*MOOTRA*)   55
- STOOLS (*PURISHA*)   55

WASTE PRODUCTS OF THE BODY

WASTE PRODUCTS (THREE *MALA*)

The three waste products of the body are the end products of digestion. They are

- Sweat (*Sweda*)
- Urine (*Mutra*)
- Stools (*Purisha*)

The food and water after absorption in the body will be excreted in the form of solid and liquid.

The solid form is in the form of stools and urine in the form of liquid.

Sweat is the waste product excreted from the body.

SWEAT (*SWEDA*)

- Sweat is secreted through pores in the body as a result of excessive activity and body heat.
- The Sweat is increased when *Pitha dosha* is increased.
- The excretion of sweat is necessary.
- But when the quantity is increased or decreased then it is alarming and requires treatment.

Reasons for abnormalities in *Sweda*

- When the person indulges in excessive activities, exposes to sunlight, extreme environment simultaneously, increased hot, sharp, sour, pungent food stuffs.
- All these activities lead to increase of *Pitha dosha* and thus produce excess sweat.

Increased Sweda

- Increased sweating, foul/bad smell from body, itchy skins are the symptoms of increased sweat production in the body.

Decreased Sweda

- Loosening of hair follicles stiff hairs and cracks in the skin (dry skin) are symptoms seen when sweat production is decreased.
- Measures that maintain increased sweat production:
- Foods which cool and maintain the body temperature are to be consumed.
- Water melon, pomegranate, grapes, pears, cucumber, lemon, ash gourd, like sandal wood dipped in water, Indian sarsaparilla are also very useful.
- Avoid food such as spicy (pepper, chilly, garlic), fried items, junk and excessive exposure to sunlight.

Measures that normalizes the reduced sweat production

- Sudation therapy
- Applications of hot body paste that activates the blocked pores in the body and makes it perspire.

URINE (*MOOTRA*)

- Urine is the waste that is excreted from the renal system.
- The color of urine ranges from little yellow to pale yellow.

Reasons for abnormalities in *Mootra*

- When a person takes more liquid diet than one needs, it causes increased urine output.

Increased urine production

- Pricking or cramping pain in the site of bladder, increased urge of micturition, feeling of non-passage of urine even after passing urine are seen.

Decreased urine output

- When the urge of micturition is withheld or less intake of water, it causes obstructed or reduced urine output.
- Decreased urine production causes decreased urine output, difficulty to pass urine, abnormal color of the urine, or blood mixed with urine.

Measures that maintain the flow of urine

- Food like barley, sugarcane juice, water, and horse gram are to be eaten.

STOOLS (*PURISHA*)

- Stools are the waste product as a result of food intake.
- The stools are solid in nature.

Reasons for abnormalities in stools

- Intake of heavy, oily, pungent, sour, salty food before digestion of previous meals.
- Indigestion, fear, anger, nervousness all this condition leads to hampered digestive fire and as a result leading to increased stool formation.
- Here *Pitha* and *Kapha doshas* are imbalanced.

Increased stools formation

- Bloating of abdomen, distension of abdomen, heaviness and colicky pain are the conditions seen.
- When there is excessive intake of dry lentils, baked items and activities like travel, excessive exercise, depression, and anxiety it leads to reduced or constipated stools.

Decreased stools formation

- Gurgling sound in intestine, colicky pain, discomfort in upper region of chest near the heart, and thorax region are seen.

Measures that maintain the stools quantity when output is increased

- Food which is sweet/sour, fibrous which increases the bulk of stools like green leafy vegetables like amaranth, spinach, kale, broccoli, green beans, carrot, barley are to be taken.
- Dairy products like milk, yogurt, also helps in easy passage of stools.

Measures that maintain the stools quantity when output is decreased

- Food with tastes bitter, astringent would reduce the increased output of stools.

AGNI

- INTRODUCTION TO *AGNI*   59
- TYPES OF *AGNI*   59
- FUNCTIONS OF *AGNI*   62
- DISEASES CAUSED BY DISTURBED *AGNI* AND ITS MANAGEMENT   62

AGNI

INTRODUCTION TO *AGNI*

- *Agni* is the most important component of the body.
- Every function of the body is dependent on the *Agni*.
- *Agni* means the fire.
- But *Agni* in our body is digestive fire.
- When *Agni* is functioning normally, the body is in healthy state.
- *Agni* is responsible for digestion.

TYPES OF *AGNI*

Agni is classified into 3 main divisions.

    1. *Jatargni*

    2. *Dhatvagni*

    3. *Bhutagni*

Jatargni

- Jatara means stomach.
- The *Agni* (digestive fire) which resides mainly in the stomach, as well as duodenum.

- This *Agni* is responsible for the taste of food, appetite, digestion as well as metabolism of food and proper elimination of waste products.

Types

A *Vishamagni*

B *Tikshnagni*

C *Mandagni*

D *Samagni*

A Vishamagni

- *Vishamagni* is the *Agni* which is irregular or variable in nature.
- It is more influenced by *Vata dosha*.
- It is has episodes of strong and weak appetite.
- In this type of *Agni* there are increased chances of having issues like abdominal pain, gas, bloating of abdomen, sour belching, sometimes loose stools and sometimes constipation.

B Tikshnagni

- *Tikshnagni* means *Agni* which is high intense or more.
- It is influenced by *Pitha dosha*.
- Here the person will have increased appetite and feel hungry soon.
- He consumes a lot of quantity of food and his digestive capacity will be very good.

C Mandagni

- *Mandagni* means Agni which is dull or low.
- It is influenced by *Kapha dosha*.
- Here the person will have very low appetite.

- The person will have poor digestive capacity and eats very less quantity of food.
- The person will have lack of taste, indigestion, nausea.

D Samagni

- *Samagni* means *agni* which is in equilibrium.
- It has all *doshas (Vata, Pitha, Kapha)* in normal/equilibrium.
- The person will have a good appetite and good digestive capacity.
- He won't be having any problems related to digestion or constipation or loose stools.

Dhatvagni

The *dhatwagni* are seven in no corresponding to the seven tissues of the body,

- They are *Rasadhatvagni (Rasa dhatu), Raktadhatvagni (Rakta dhatu), Mamsadhatvagni (Mamsa dhatu), Meda dhatvagni (Meda dhatu), Asthi dhatvagni (Asthi dhatu), Majja dhatvagni (Majja dhatu), Shukra dhatvagni (Shukra dhatu)*.
- These *Agni* nourishes corresponding tissues and helps in the normal functions.

Bhutagni

Bhutagni are five in number.

- They are *Parthiva agni* (Earth element), *Apya agni* (Water element), *Teja agni* (Fire element), *Vayavya agni* (Wind element), *Nabhasa agni* (Space element).
- Each *Agni* resides in corresponding *mahabhutas* (5 elements).

FUNCTIONS OF *AGNI*

- *Agni* is not only responsible for digestion of the food but also for the proper elimination of waste products.
- The food what we eat is digested by *Agni* and later separated as nutrient part and waste part.
- The nutrient part nourishes all the tissues, the 3 *Doshas* as well as the whole body.
- While waste part is completely eliminated in the form of sweat, urine and stools.

DISEASES CAUSED BY DISTURBED *AGNI* AND ITS MANAGEMENT

- Diseases are caused due to disturbed digestive fire.
- The disturbance can be in terms of low and increased digestive fire.
- Low digestive fire leads to conditions such as lack of taste, lack of appetite, indigestion, Constipation, gas.
- High digestive fire leads to increased appetite, burning sensation, mouth ulcer, loose stools, Irritable bowel syndrome, Acidity.
- Low digestive fire should be managed by intake of appetizers and give warm light food.
- Avoid heavy food such as curds, milk, meat, cheese.
- One should take cumin water, ginger water, soups, steamed food, fruits like pomegranate, orange etc.
- High digestive fire should be managed by normalizing the increased digestive fire.

- One should consume food which is having qualities like cold, sweet, heavy.
- One should take food like milk, ghee, butter, steamed banana, rice, sweets.

THREE PILLARS OF LIFE

- FOOD — 67
- DESCRIPTION ABOUT EACH TASTE
  (CHARACTERISTICS, ACTION, EFFECTS OF OVERUSE) — 68
- TIME OF FOOD INTAKE — 82
- DIETETIC RULES — 82
- ANTAGONISTIC FOOD (*VIRUDDHARA*) — 85
- TYPES OF ANTAGONISTIC FOOD — 85
- SLEEP — 89
- *HOMA* THERAPY — 96
- THIRTEEN NATURAL URGES THAT IS NOT BE CONTROLLED — 97

THREE PILLARS OF LIFE

1. Food
2. Sleep
3. Life style/Ethics

- The three main pillars of life are Food, Sleep, Behavioral aspects.
- It acts like pillars for the human body.
- If any one of these is disturbed, then the body tends to be weaker, divergent from the health.
- Insufficient, excess, improper habits of these three gives rise to many health problems.

FOOD

Refer Fig 1.3

- There is a good saying that "A man is what he eats."
- The food nourishes the body and is an essential factor for life.
- The food we eat is partly assimilated in the body and partly eliminated as waste product through sweat, urine, and feces.
- When food is eaten qualitatively, quantitatively and in a proper manner it acts as nectar whereas, if not it becomes toxic to the body.
- Thus it causes disturbance in three *doshas* and seven tissues in the body resulting in diseases.
- There are various factors that should be taken care of while eating food.
- Food relishes the taste buds.

Thus food will be made of different tastes, six tastes namely:

1. Sweet
2. sour
3. salty
4. spicy
5. bitter, and
6. astringent.

- When all the tastes are taken in proper quantities, it will lead to good health.
- If only one particular taste is taken daily it would imbalance the three *doshas* and leads to disease.

DESCRIPTION ABOUT EACH TASTE (CHARACTERISTICS, ACTION, EFFECTS OF OVERUSE)

SWEET

- Sweet taste is made up of earth and water elements.

Qualities

- Sweet is the most relishing among all six tastes.
- When sweet taste comes into contact with the tongue, it forms a coating in the mouth and brings about pleasant feelings to body and mind.
- Ants are attracted to the sweetness of food.

Actions

- Sweet taste is wholesome to the body, provides strength to the body tissues.
- This taste is beneficial to children, old, injured, lean, promotes complexion, hair growth, and provides strength to the sense organs.

Benefits

- It is nutritious, smoothens the voice, increases the breast milk, and heals the cells, heavy in nature.
- Consumption of sweet in limited quantity provides long life span, smoothness, pacifies *Pitha-Vata dosha,* anti-toxic.

Examples

- Vegetables: pumpkin, sweet potato, beetroot, carrot, ash gourd.
- Fruits: Banana, grapes, cherries, ripened mango, apple, chikku, dates, and raisins.
- Milk, ghee, or honey, sugarcane juice, Sugar, jaggery, rice, coconut.

Ayurveda medicine

Kushmanda rasayana

- It provides nourishment to the body especially in loss of body weight.

Chyavanaprasha

- It builds up the immunity, antioxidant, and vitality, cures cough, asthma.

Narasimha rasayana

- It is best medicine for initiating hair growth and strengthening the roots of hair. Better to be avoided in person with *Pitha* predominance and *Pitha* related disorders.
- It increases male characteristics; it should be taken in caution by women.

Side effects of overuse

Excessive use of sweet causes increase in fat tissue, *Kapha* diseases like Obesity, reduced digestive fire, altered consciousness, Diabetes, Goitre, Tumors.

SOUR

Sour taste is made up of fire and earth element.

Qualities

- When the sour taste comes into contact with the mouth it cleanses the mouth by its sharp action.
- It causes goose bumps, increases the sensitivity of teeth, and causes a sudden contraction of eyebrows and eyes.

Actions

- It increases the digestive fire, and increases the taste perception.
- It is hot in quality, cold to touch, nourishing and light for digestion.

Benefits

- Sour taste brings pleasantness to the body and mind; hence it is good for heart.
- It increases *Kapha* and *Pitha doshas* and increases circulation.

Examples

- Tomato, tamarind, cocum, yoghurt, pomegranate, fermented drinks, buttermilk.
- Ayurveda medicines like

§ *Dadimadi ghrita*

- It corrects digestion, increases blood count, and cures Irritable bowel disease, helpful in curing female infertility.

§ *Chinchadi lehya*
- It cures Piles, Constipation, Anemia and Jaundice.

§ *Changeriyadi ghrita*
- It cures Gastritis, Piles and Hyperacidity.

Side effects of overuse
- Excessive use of sour taste causes wrinkling of skin, reduced eyes sight, and reduced consciousness.
- Skin itching, paleness, swelling of body, blisters, thirst, increased body temperature (Hyperthermia).

SALTY
- Salty taste is made up of water and fire elements.

Qualities
- Food having salty taste when comes in contact with the mouth, causes watering of the mouth, slight irritation in oral cavity and throat.

Action
- It increases the digestive fire, causes sweating because of its sharp nature, provides taste to the food, abrasive in action, piercing.

Examples
- Natural salt, black salt, sea salt.

Side effects of overuse
- When consumed in excess it vitiates and increases *rakta-vata*, premature greying and hair fall, and wrinkling of skin, thirst, skin diseases, cellulitis, toxins, reduces the body strength.

SPICY

- Spicy taste is made up of fire and air elements.

Qualities

- When food having spicy taste comes in contact with the taste buds it causes piercing or strong effect on tip of the tongue.
- It also causes watering of the eyes, nose, and mouth as it increases the sensation of taste buds.

Actions

- It increases the digestion, improves the appetite, cleans up the body channels, disintegrates blocks or obstructions, and pacifies the *Kapha dosha*.

Benefits

- It cures the diseases of throat, skin diseases, Urticaria.
- It helps in digesting the toxic stagnated food in stomach,
- It reduces swelling, dries up smoothness, moisture, mucous, lipids of body.

Examples

- Chilly, pepper, garlic, spices like cinnamon, asafetida, ginger, cow urine.

§ *Talisapatradi choorna*

- It is medicine with spices like pepper, used in respiratory condition where there is consolidation of mucus.

§ *Trikatu choorna*

- It is made up of three spices which have spicy taste; advised to correct poor digestive fire.

Side effects of overuse

- When spicy food is consumed in excess it causes thirst, loss of sexual drive, loss of strength, muscle cramps, imbalance in consciousness, tremors, aching pain in the hip and back regions etc.

BITTER

- Bitter taste is made up of space and air elements.

Qualities

- Bitter taste is light, dry and cold by nature.

Actions

- When it comes in contact with the tongue, it tastes bad.

Benefits

- Bitter taste manages to cure loss of appetite, worm infestations, thirst, toxicity, altered consciousness.
- It is effective in Fever, skin ailments, increased mucous secretion and burning sensation.
- It pacifies *Pitha* and *Kapha doshas*, but causes drying up of the mucous, lipids, fats, bone marrow, urine, feces.
- It promotes intelligence, cleans throat, and purifies breast milk.

Examples

- Bitter gourd, amaranth leaves, fenugreek, neem, snake gourd etc.
- Ayurvedic medicines like

§ *Tikta ghrita*

- It is basically very bitter but has excellent results in skin diseases like Psoriasis, Eczema, and weight loss.

§ *Guggulu tikta ghrita*

- It is very bitter in taste yet very effective in reducing high cholesterol levels, Psoriatic Arthritis, and weight loss.

Side effects of overuse

- When taken in excess it causes depletion of body tissues and diseases related to Vata dosha aggravation.

Refer Fig 1.4

ASTRINGENT

- Astringent taste is made up of earth and air elements.

Action

- When foods having astringent taste come in contact with the taste buds, it makes the tongue heavier and constricts the throat.

Benefits

- The astringent taste pacifies *Kapha* and *Pitha doshas*.
- It is heavy, purifies the blood, promotes healing and is cold in nature.
- It brings down the body fat, removes the excess oiliness from skin.
- It is constipative, causes dryness and enhances the skin tone.
- Eg: legumes, unripened fruits of lemon, ficus, pearl, dates when unripened.
- Ayurveda herbs like
    1. *Haritaki (Terminalia chebula), Vibhitaki (Terminalia bellirica), Khadira (Acacia catechu).*

Side effects of overuse

- When consumed in excess causes distress in the abdomen, pain in chest region, weight loss, loss in sex drive, obstruction in channels and Constipation.

Refer Fig 1.5

There are certain rules that are to be followed while eating

- Food what we eat is the main contributor for our life.
- Food is the main reason for health.

Few things if followed while eating would contribute maximum benefits to the body in terms of

- Strengthening the body both physically and mentally
- Nourishment of the body
- Proper functioning of the senses
- Good voice
- Good complexion
- Happiness
- Satisfaction
- Enthusiasm
- Memory

Proper time for food intake

§ Timing of the food should be given prime importance. If time is not given importance, then the food what we eat will turn to be the cause of illness.

§ One should take food when one has the following

- When a person has clear belching
- Enthusiasm
- Proper movement of urine stools.
- Initiation of thirst and hunger

§ If all these are felt then it is the right time to have food.

Order of Food intake

- One should first take sweet food as it increases salivation and helps in proper chewing.
- One should eat when hungry.
- Intake of food like spicy, salty in the beginning would have ill effects on the digestive system.
- Whereas food having sweet taste is taken first, it strengthens the mucous membrane of the digestive system making it healthy and strong.
- Sour and salty food should be taken next, so that one can appreciate the taste of food.
- One can't imagine any food to be tasty without salt in it.
- Pungent, bitter food should be taken lastly as it helps in the absorption, proper digestion of the fat and heavy contents in the food.
- It makes the digestion lighter and provides comfort after the meal.

Eight criteria of healthy food

- Natural quality
- Processing
- Combination

- Quantity
- Habitat
- Time
- Dietetic rules
- User

§ In order to gain maximum benefits of food, knowledge of all criteria's above should be considered before eating.

§ By following this there will be maximum benefits on health, one can know various factors like which is good for one's body and which is not.

§ What time to eat and how to eat, what quantity to eat, if over eaten how it affects the digestion activity and many factors that will lead to qualitative life.

Natural qualities

- Natural quality is inbuilt nature of the food.
- Few are light whereas few are heavy.
- Few are dry whereas few are unctuous.

Examples

Green gram: it is very light easily digested when cooked properly,.

- It is good to eliminate excess *Kapha dosha*, good in Diabetic patients and Obesity.

Black gram: basically very heavy, digested with difficulty.

- People with poor digestive fire cannot digest easily giving rise to indigestion.
- Peas/chana are very dry and light in nature which aggravates *Vata dosha*, if eaten in excess will lead to gastric troubles.

- Meat of pork, buffalo is very unctuous and heavy which aggravates *Kapha dosha*.

Processing

- Processing of food brings alteration to its natural qualities.
- This alteration takes place when mixed with water, cooked with heat, added with flavors, preservation with various substances.
- Eg: Rice which is heavy when processed into parched rice is lighter to digest.
- The powder of roasted grains when fried, makes different preparations turns heavy.

Food combination

- Food combination means mixing two or more products.
- Thus it exhibits a third property due to a combination which is very powerful.
- Example: Milk only is nourishing, but when mixed with required proportion of water and garlic paste would act to remove excess fat or cholesterol from the body.

Quantity

- Quantity is another important entity to maintain health.
- Anything in limit provides benefits to health whereas anything in more will act as toxins.
- Similarly in food, there is food with different properties as told above.
- Heavy food like black gram should be taken $1/3^{rd}$ or ½ the capacity of a individual.
- Food like green gram having lighter quality should be eaten in more quantity.

- According to Ayurveda it is told that half of the stomach should be filled by solid food, quarter by liquid food and the remaining free space for air to ensure proper digestion.
- If food is taken in low quantity it affects the body with loss of strength, reduced bodyweight and virility, impaired functions in the body.
- If taken in large quantity it is said to aggravate all the doshas and lead to indigestion, Obesity etc.

Habitat

- The habitat is variable.
- Specific food is available in specific habitat.
- It also depends on the nature of the soil, climate and other factors.
- There are three types of habitat according to Ayurveda,
    1. Wild/dry/forest
    2. Marshy
    3. Moderate/normal

Wild/dry/forest area

- Dry or wild area has very deep and thick forest.
- Soil will be very fertile and black, red or whitish colour.
- The water availability here will be very less.
- Big trees are found.
- Crops like green gram, dal etc. grows here.
- Animals like lion, tiger, camel, sheep, horse and buffalo are found.
- People residing here will have more of dry nature i.e. *Vata dosha* properties.
- They will be thin, having dry skin, strong and rough body.

- If person takes more of dry, light or cold property food, he will suffer from debility, loss of weight, neurological problems, and dry skin.
- So nutritious food like milk products, sweet, sour food are to be taken.
- Eg: middle part of India like Africa, Tibet, and Mongolia.
- Food of these countries like Africa should consume food more of unctuous, sharp, and hot qualities in order to reduce the increased *Vata dosha*.
- I.e. milk products, meat products, starchy food, grilled meat sausages, spinach stew cooked with tomato, pepper, onion, peanut and butter.
- Fat rich food like ghee, yogurt, milk products, coconut and sweet are to be consumed.

Marshy land

- In marshy lands adequate water is available and lands will be covered with mud.
- Small grass, bushes, creepers, and greenery will be seen all over.
- The land is surrounded by green forests, green creeper covered mountains.
- Cold wind keeps circulating.
- The land has ponds with water and beautiful lotus, lily.
- Black gram, sugarcane, mango, jackfruit, coconut trees are mainly seen.
- People residing in this area will have well-nourished body or over weight, fair skin, delicate body.
- Here diseases mainly of *Kapha dosha* are seen.
- Food which sweet, unctuous, heavy are to be avoided.

- If taken would cause diseases like increased cholesterol, diabetes, obesity, skin problems.
- Foods having light, sharp qualities, bitter, astringent taste food are to be taken to maintain equilibrium.

Examples

- Himalayan foot hills, parts of Europe, northern America.
- Himalayan region: wheat bread or roti, maize, barley, millet.
- Fruits like lemon, mangoes, Asian pear.
- European region: more of beetroot soup, bread, meats, cheese, variety of wines.
- Northern America: steak, grilled meat, shrimp, burrito, tacos, buffalo meat, wild turkey meat, sweets like Apple pie, use of spices like nutmeg, ginger, cinnamon, cloves, black pepper.

Normal land

- Environmental conditions in this land will be normal or moderate.
- Soil color here is red to white.
- Climate is neither too dry nor too moist.
- There will be neither cold or hot wind nor not much rain.
- It has moderate season.
- In normal land there won't be any variation in *doshas*.
- People here always remain healthy.
- Eg: Mediterranean, Central India, and Central America.
- Mediterranean food: olive, grape, wheat, olive oil, garlic, local pungent wine, figs, basil, apricot.
- Central Indian food: wheat, rice, fish.
- Here wide variety of food can be taken as the climate is favorable for almost all kinds of food as it has moderate type of climate.

TIME OF FOOD INTAKE

- Time is another main factor for food.
- Time if followed properly will yield excellent health in the body.
- The best time to eat food is after complete digestion of previous meals, when a person gets hungry.
- The minimum is to give three hours of gap between meals.

Meals are to be taken according to season

- A good quantity of food can be taken for breakfast and mid-day meal.
- Light and less quantity of food should be taken in the evening preferably before 7–7:30 pm (19–19:30 hours).
- During the day time the digestive fire will be high, so one can digest heavy quantity of food.
- In the night the digestive fire will be milder, with less capacity to digest.
- If one takes heavy food in the evening hours, it results in indigestion or hampers the digestive fire on the long run.

DIETETIC RULES

- There are certain rules and limitations for any kind of work to have a good result, similarly the food.
- If food is eaten in a systematic way, the body will benefit.

Eat warm/hot food

- Warm or hot food stimulates the digestive fire, and enhances the taste buds.
- Warm food thus helps in the downward movement of air in the alimentary tract resulting in comfort of body.
- Eating warm food regulates or checks profuse flow of saliva and gastric juices.

Eat unctuous food

- Eating unctuous food ensures the proper flow of air in the alimentary tract and an increase in the digestive fire.
- It is similar as if when ghee is poured on fire, it burns with a high flame.
- Unctuous food enhances early digestion, nourishes the body, strengthens the sense organs and increases complexion.

Eat right amount of food

- A person should never eat to his full capacity.
- Half of the stomach should be filled by solid food, quarter by liquid food and the remaining free space for air to ensure proper digestion.
- If a person eats proper quantity of food one feels light, energetic.
- There will be no distress in the stomach, no heaviness in the chest region and the sense organs function properly.
- Other benefits would be an ease in doing activities like walking, standing, sitting, breathing.
- It also imparts good strength, digestion, and complexion.

Eat only after the digestion of previous meals

- Food is to be always eaten after experiencing features like:
- Reappearance of hunger, secretion of gastric juices, clear belching, normal peristaltic movements, evacuation of urine, stools, flatus.
- Then it serves the purpose or benefit of having food.
- A person if takes food prior to digestion of the previous meals it will cause indigestion of food.

Eat food articles that are not of opposite/antagonistic potency

- Each food has specific properties.
- Few combination of food will be beneficial, whereas few would harm the equilibrium of *Doshas* ending up with ill health.
- Eg: curd and fish have two different potencies, curd being cool and fish being hot.
- If taken together this will cause various ill effects on the skin, body, and digestion.
- Whereas curds with sugar is a good combination since both are having cold potency.
- It benefits the body.

Eat in the right place

- Eating in a right place and place of choice with all necessary equipment would have a positive and pleasant impact on body and mind.
- Maintenance of hygiene, devoid of dirt or places of cremation, unwanted people are to be avoided.

Never eat too fast

- If food is taken fast, it has the chances to enter the respiratory tract causing aspiration.
- If taken fast have chances of increasing *Vata dosha* thus affecting digestion.

Never eat too slowly

- If food is eaten very slow, there will be less satisfaction to the body.
- The food thus loses its temperature and becomes cold and hampers the digestion.

Don't speak, laugh while eating and eat with concentration

- One, who laughs, speaks while eating, faces the same difficulties as those who eat too fast.
- Food should be taken wholeheartedly with full concentration so as to keep the mind calm and enjoy the food.

Eat according to the constitution of the body

- Persons should eat according to their body nature, digestion power, and wholesomeness.
- People of *Vata dosha* constitution if eats more dry, light food it affects one's digestion or nutrition.
- One should eat heavier, unctuous, hot food.

ANTAGONISTIC FOOD (*VIRUDDHARA*)

- There are certain food substances which are opposite (antagonistic) in nature, which when consumed in combination leads to adverse effects on health.
- When it is taken knowingly or unknowingly, comes in contact with digestive fire.
- It forms a product which is difficult to digest or being absorbed by body, forms toxins (*Ama*).
- Thus it causes adverse effects on the body and mind.

TYPES OF ANTAGONISTIC FOOD

1 Food antagonistic for place

- In dry places like dessert already having dry nature the hot atmosphere; eating drier, hot substances like horse gram, spicy pickles.

- In places like coastal area where atmosphere is unctuous; eating more heavy and unctuous food substances like black gram, curds, sweets, fried items.
- It causes toxins in the body giving rise to various health issues.

2 Food antagonistic to season

- In season like winter if one eats more of cold and dry food substances like eating cereals and pulses like peas, Chick peas (*chana*), lentils, cold water intake.

3 Food antagonistic to digestive fire

- If digestive fire is medium and then person eats very heavy food like curds, milk of buffalo.

4 Food antagonistic to quantity

- Ghee and honey are the ones which when taken in same quantity would lead to toxins in the body.

5 Food antagonistic to wholesomeness

- If a person always sweet food and he suddenly tends to eat sour substance.
- It causes antagonistic food effect in body.

6 Food antagonistic to *Dosha*

- If a person having predominant *Kapha dosha* consumes heavier, unctuous, sweet food like curds, sweets, sugar, and oily food, it is antagonistic.

7 Food antagonistic while processing

- Curds when heated or honey when heated turns into toxins.

8 Food antagonistic to one's digestive system

- **People with dry or hard stools if they eat or drink** very less food, dry food, less water like lentils, green gram, peas, chapatti is an example.

9 Food antagonistic to potency

- Intake of food having cold potency along with hot potency.
- Like yogurt and milk (cold potency) if taken with fish (hot potency) would be antagonistic.

Refer Fig 1.6

10 Food antagonistic to situation

- When a person is tired after exposure to sun/heat and he suddenly eats or drink chilled food is an example.

11 Food antagonistic to sequence

- If a person takes food before having strong appetite or remaining hungry for long time.

12 Food antagonistic to treatment

- If a person is not advised to take heavy products like milk products or egg during *Panchakarma* treatment like *Snehapana* (ghee therapy) and if he still eats it.

13 Food antagonistic to cooking

- If food is over cooked or over fried (burnt) or undercooked.

14 Food antagonistic to combination

- Intake of milk while eating banana or taking sour substance with milk.

15 Food antagonistic to interest

- Intake of food which is unpleasant or unhygienic, in unhygienic environment.

16 Food antagonistic to quality or richness

- Eating a fruit which is unripened or over ripened or stale.

17 Food antagonistic to rules of eating

Taking meals while speaking or laughing or in a crowded place with noise.

Common examples like

- Mixing honey with hot water.
- Curd at night.
- Cold water after hot coffee.
- Combination of milk and fruits.
- Meat cooked with curd or heating curds.
- Fish and milk combination.

- Antagonistic food in the body.
- Antagonistic food is like a foreign particle or reaction in body which triggers immune system as a response to foreign pathogens, histamine is produced in the body.

Histamine produced by the mast cells, to help the body deal with irritation caused by allergens or foreign bodies.

The histamine released causes allergic symptoms, these release can be deadly too.

When the histamine reaches the site it causes effects like dilation of small blood vessels known as inflammatory response or swelling.

It results in Urticaria.

It also causes constriction of smooth muscles, affects the bronchi muscles in respiratory system and breathing gets difficult.

Increased vascular permeability causes fluid to escape from the capillaries into the tissue which leads to running nose and watering in the eyes.

Histamines suppress the gastric acid secretion, thus reduce the appetite and has effect on sleep. Thus, causing insomnia.

SLEEP

- Sleep is the second major part of life. Without sleep it's impossible to have a comfortable day.
- The sleep is a essential phenomenon similar to water and food which restores energy when practiced in a proper way.

Causes of sleep

- Increased *Kapha dosha*.
- Increased dullness in mind. (*Tamoguna*)
- Increased exhaustion (mind and body)
- Natural cause/by habit

The quality in body and mind responsible for sleep is *Kapha dosha* and dull mind.

When these are altered, there will be either less or excessive sleep which in turn leads to diseases.

When the mind and body is surrounded by dull mind and *Kapha dosha*, the person falls asleep.

It is the state of sub consciousness where the sense organs detach contact with their senses and enter into a phenomenon called sleep.

Sleep according to *Doshas*

Sleep for Persons with *Vata dosha*

- The people of this nature sleep less, as there is more dryness and alertness.
- The sleep quality will be poor.
- The persons of this nature wakes up even with small sound.

Sleep for Persons with *Pitha dosha*

- The people of this nature sleep moderately, more alert.
- The quality of sleep will be moderate.
- They fall asleep very early and wake up early too.

Sleep for Persons with *Kapha dosha*

- The person of this nature sleeps for a long time.
- The quality of sleep will be very high.

- They fall asleep very soon and wake up very late.
- The deepest sounds do not wake him.

Few ill sleeping habits
- Sleeping late night.
- Sleeping till late in the morning.
- Sleeping during the day.
- Sleeping soon after food.
- Sleeping on improper surface or improper position (like prone, with legs upper than the body level or with head lower than body level).
- Eating very heavy food before sleeping.
- Sleeping in places which are haunted or unhygienic, near water bodies, damp places, places where animals reside.

Improper sleep effects
- Sleep is one of the three pillars of life.
- If one pillar is not strong in a building, then the whole building gets collapsed.
- Sleeplessness or reduced sleep causes discomfort in all ways and affect both the body and mind equally.

Effects of improper sleep
- Improper sleep leads to poor attention, poor concentration, Depression, forgetfulness, lethargic, confusion, altered consciousness.
- Inability to make decisions, Anxiety, lack of confidence, mental illness like Schizophrenia, Attention Deficit Hyperactivity syndrome.

- Visual impairment reduced hearing, heart disease, High blood pressure, Stroke, Diabetes, loss of sex drive, skin aging, weight gain or loss, hormonal imbalance.

Ayurveda has beautifully and logically explained the treatment for reduced sleep or insomnia

- Oil massage – both head and full body massage with *Bala ashwagandha* oil, *Ksirabala* oil.
- Head massage with *Himasagara* oil, *Brahmi* oil, *Chandanadi* oil.
- Foot massage – it improves circulation to brain and promotes good sleep.
- Eg: *kshira bala* oil, *Narayana* oil.
- Instillation of nasal drops with *Kshira bala* oil.
- Paste on the head like *Jatamamsi, Vacha*.

§ Therapies like *Shirodhara* (pouring of stream of oil on forehead), *Shirovasti* (retention of oil on the scalp), retention of medicated ghee in the eyes, bathing.

§ Green leafy vegetables like ash guard, pumpkin, sweet potato, bottle guard, tomatoes, and broccoli are to be taken.

§ Fruits like banana, cherries, papaya, pineapple and watermelon.

§ Milk, fermented beverages, meat, curd should be consumed.

§ Dry fruits like walnut, raisins.

§ Black gram, rice, wheat, ragi.

§ Milk and milk products like ghee, butter, cottage cheese, lassi.

§ Fish and meat like mutton, beef, pork and turkey.

Measures to be taken in the case of excess sleep

- Procedure like emesis, collyriums and nasal drops with strong and sharp medicine are to be done.
- Patient should be subjected to fasting therapy.
- One should do excess thinking, grief, anger, and sexual activities.
- All these bring down the *Kapha dosha* and reduce the excess sleep.
- Activities like Yoga, pranayama or sports.
- Yoga like *Janu-Shirsasana, Baddhakonasana, Balasana, Marjarasana, Shavasana, Yoga Nidra.*
- *Pranayama* like *Nadishudhi, Sheetali, Sitkari.*
- One should indulge in sports like cricket, tennis, swimming, walking, cycling, and jogging.
- Avoid heavy meals at night; one should have dinner by 8:30 pm.
- Avoid long conversations at night.
- Avoid t.v, cell phones, and laptops while sleeping.

Effects of proper sleep

- Just imagine your day without previous night sleep. How tiring, uneasy, it would be?
- The symptoms of proper sleep are pleasantness, happiness, nourishment, strength, vigor, knowledge, ability to concentrate, vitality, good and long life.
- Thus balancing all the *doshas* of the body and mind.
- Hence sleep is responsible for a wonderful health and life.

Abstinence (Life style or Ethics) to be followed in a society

- The soul meaning of abstinence is not just being away from sex or sexual desires.
- It means being closer to the wisdom or the right knowledge, also the right age for certain rituals in life.
- The body as well as the mind does not attain enough maturity to take responsibility and reproduce up to the age of 25 years in men and 18 years in women.
- In case the boy or girl involve in sexual act before the age limit, the body becomes weak like the juice extracted from unripen mango.
- The body strength, body tissues, vitality all decreases soon and the child born will have birth defects or weaker strength according to Ayurveda.
- According to Ayurveda, the sexual related problems and treatment is discussed under *Vasti* and useful topic called *Vajeekarana* (aphrodisiac/ one which increases the sexual drive).
- The semen of the man is said to be the end product of all the six tissues, hence it has to be taken care.

Few behavioral aspects followed in day to day life

- The society to be peaceful, every individual is responsible.
- If an individual follows few ethics and mannerisms, then he himself will be happy, pleasant.
- Hence he contributes to the society positively.
- Comfort in our lives is utmost importance to us.
- Yes, it is obvious for a happy life.

- There are certain things along with our comforts which we need to think about and beyond.
- If things around us are happy and healthy, naturally it would add up to our comfort and happiness.
- *Dharma* (virtue) is the one which gives utmost comfort providing.
- Everybody should follow some virtues.
- In the path of virtue, there are few sins which should not be committed. i.e.
- Violence, theft, infidelity, bearing/calumny, abuse/rude, speaking lie/untruthful, uttering rubbish, tendency to harm, longing to have others belongings, atheism.
- One should help poor, sick and mentally weak and should be merciful or have sympathy towards small creatures like worms, ants etc.
- Worshiping of the God should be done daily, people like physician, scholars, guests, old people should be honored.
- Cows should be respected or adored as they are sacred.
- One who approaches for help should not be sent back disappointed, insulted or defamed.
- Envy the cause not the result.
- Way to talk or deal.
- One should always speak about relevant topics with positive attitude and pleasing way, to the point, attractively.
- Talk should be pulling people towards you like a magnet.
- Always have a good conduct, compassion pleasant behavior.
- Sharing your joy with people.
- But never trust people more than necessary nor be too susceptive.

HOMA THERAPY

- *Homa* is a Sanskrit terminology meaning ritual or religious offering made into fire.
- The other terms used for it are *Yajna, Agnihotra, and Havana.*
- Here offerings are done to the fire with substance like milk, ghee, yogurt, rice, sweets with assistance of priest.
- The fire altar (*Homa kunda*) is mainly made of brick/copper or brass metal which has square shape which is predominant of earth element.
- The wooden sticks or sandal wood sticks are again predominant of earth and the ghee poured into it is predominant of water element.
- The fire lit is predominant of fire and air elements.
- The offerings of *Tulasi,* aromatic herb stuffs like camphor and cow dung are added.

Time of this ritual

- Early in the morning 6 am or in the evening 6 pm.
- This time is chosen as the environment will have the influence of sun rays.
- The sun when it is about to rise or just after the sunset, the surroundings will be comparatively calm.

Main aim

- The life being too fast, there are too many health problems arising both physically and mentally.
- The stress arising maybe due to work or other relationships in life.
- The modern life is responsible for polluting the fresh atmosphere, where this plays an important role.

- Purification of the body, mind and atmosphere is the main intension of this therapy.

Mode of action
- The action of the *Homa* therapy can be explained with the help of the ways it is performed and ingredients used.
- Wooden sticks and the oil: produces mainly the fire element.
- Ghee: produces the oxygen that is containing the earth and water elements.
- Rice grains: acts mainly on the air element.
- Basil leaves and aromatic herbs: acts on air and space elements.
- Sweet in the form of jaggery and sugar: acts on water element.

Chemical constituents
- Formalic acid purifies the atmosphere and reduces infection.
- Acetic acid: kills the bacillus coli, prevents infection, and prevents the decaying of fruits and vegetables.
- Pyrolologenic acid: acts as antiseptic.
- Vanilic acid: antiseptic

THIRTEEN NATURAL URGES THAT IS NOT BE CONTROLLED

1. Gas in terms of flatus and belching
2. Defecation
3. Micturition
4. Sneezing

5. Thirst
6. Hunger
7. Sleep
8. Cough
9. Panting
10. Yawning
11. Crying/Lacrimation
12. Vomiting
13. Ejaculation/orgasm.

§ The natural urges if suppressed causes weakness of the body.

§ If the urge for defecation or flatus is controlled, it will give rise to stomach disturbance, bloating, digestive problems, piles, anal diseases.

§ If micturation urge is controlled it causes heaviness, pain and stones in the bladder.

§ Sneezing, cough, panting if controlled causes respiratory disorders.

§ Yawning urge if controlled causes locked jaw, pain in the cheek bones, facial muscle weakness.

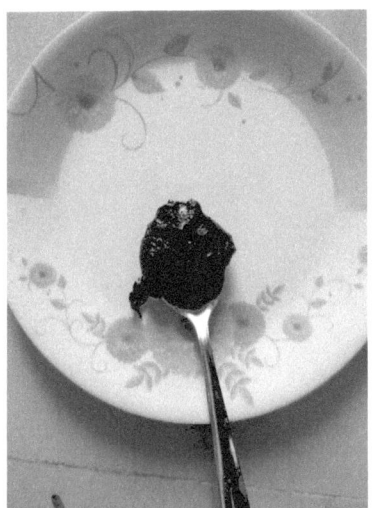
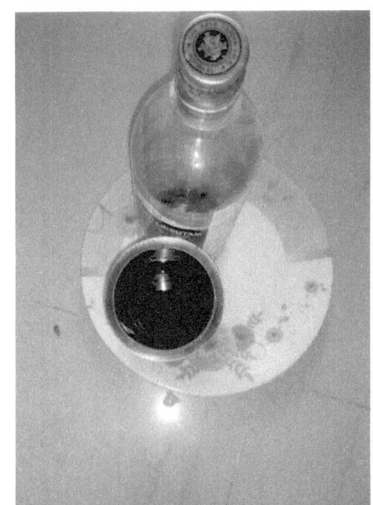
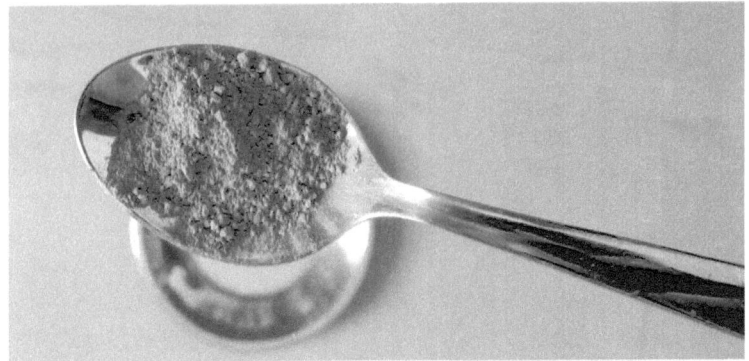

Fig 1.0 Different Forms of Medicines

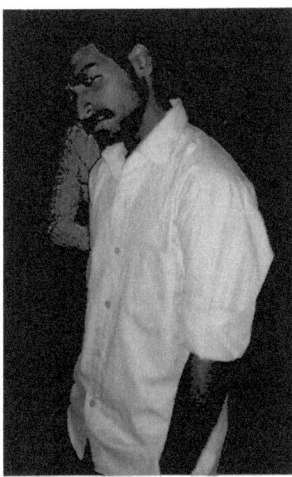
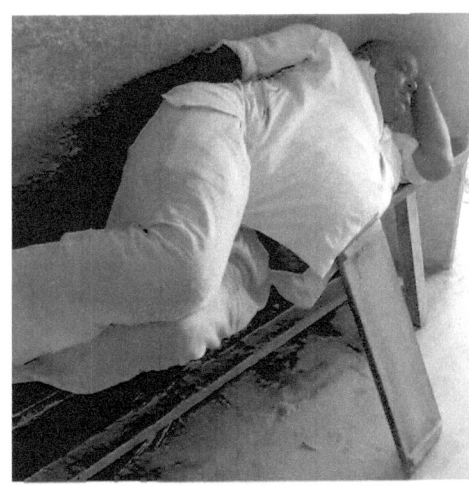

Fig 1.1 Aggresive Mind

Fig 1.2 Dull Mind

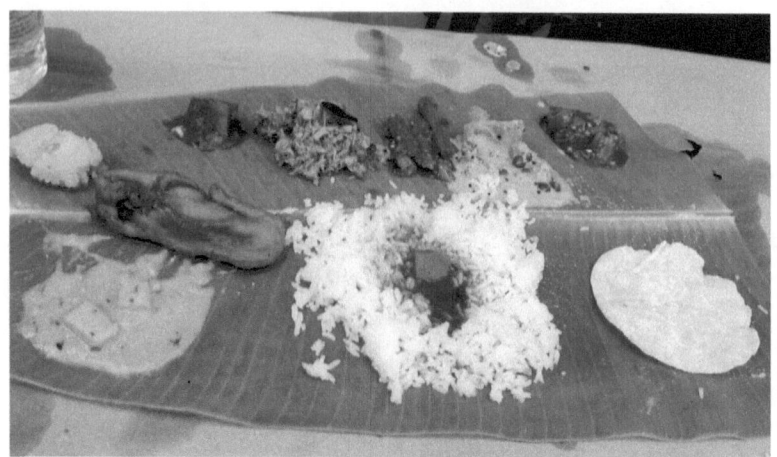

Fig 1.3 Food

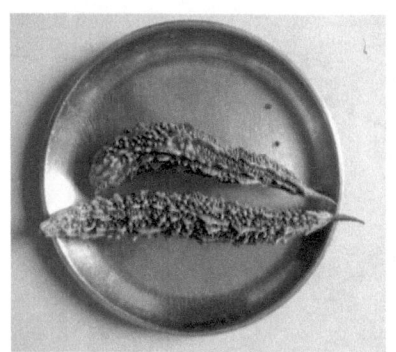

Fig 1.4 Bitter Taste

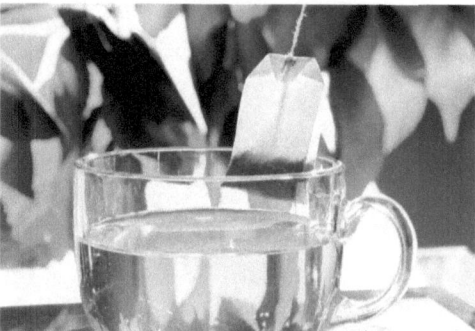

Fig 1.5 Astringent Taste

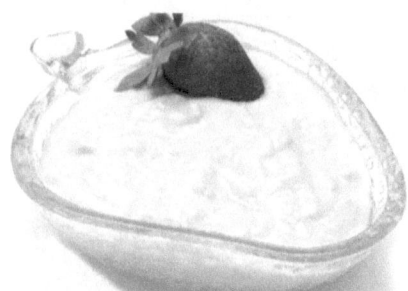
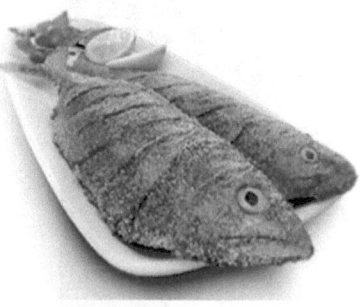

Fig 1.6 Food Antagonistic to Potency

DAILY REGIMEN

- WAKE UP TIME — 103
- BOWEL HABIT — 104
- CLEANING THE TEETH — 104
- GARGLING — 105
- NASAL DROPS — 106
- COLLYRIUM — 107
- EXERCISE — 108
- OIL MASSAGE — 111
- POWDER MASSAGE — 113
- BATH — 114
- FOOD — 115
- BODY HYGIENE — 115
- PROTECTION FROM EXTERNAL ENVIRONMENT — 116

DAILY REGIMEN (*DINACHARYA*)

- In present era people are getting too busy with their work schedule.
- They have irregular sleep timing and wake up being tired.
- The whole day is spent abruptly that there is no particular time table.
- Ayurveda has an answer for it.
- Daily regimen is told as to have a systematic life, so as to be aware of what we ourselves are doing.
- Benefits: to have a good life span, to be healthy physically and mentally.

WAKE UP TIME

- Waking up about 96 min before sunrise is best for the body, because the environment will be fresh and more oxygen is generated.
- So one can breathe more of oxygen due to which his body will be lively throughout the day.
- Mental capacity is said to be at its peak in the morning.
- People who study early in the morning will have more grasping power and ability to recollect the learnt things will be higher than other time of day.
- The mind will be optimistic, free from mental disturbances.
- There will be more creativity, intelligence.

- If one wake up early, there will be adequate time for yourself and you can plan your day well.
- In this process mind remains calm, free from stress or tension and remains pleasant and happy.
- After waking up it is always advised to pray god because it will bring energy and state of wellbeing, state for protectiveness, increased concentration power, calm mind.

BOWEL HABIT

- One should evacuate urine and stools after waking up.
- It brings lightness and liveliness of the body after evacuation of waste from body.
- Later one should clean the genital area and maintain proper hygiene.

CLEANING THE TEETH

- It is a must to brush teeth because teeth is an important one by which we can chew food and speak clearly.
- The first time we express positive attitude towards good people or greet people is smile.
- Speech is important to maintain oral hygiene. So brushing the teeth is to be done with herbs having acidic (mild), bitter, astringent taste.
- It has cleansing property as it scraps out the deposited plaque, increases the shine and maintains the normal color of teeth.
- A soft brush is preferred. After every meal a person can clean his teeth.

- Using taste like sweet, salty, sour will hamper the enamel of teeth and bring about increased sensitivity in teeth.
- Eg: paste containing *Nimba or Neem* (*Azadirachta indica*), *Khadira* (*Acascia catechu*), *Yashtimadhu* or Liquorice (*Glycyrrhiza glabra*), *Lavanga* or Clove powder (*Syzygium aromaticum*) etc.

GARGLING

- Water or medicated decoction or liquid, oil, milk is put into mouth and kept (with movement or without movement) is called Gargling.
- It is also called oil pulling therapy.
- It is done in order to have an oral hygiene, reduce or eliminate the diseases of mouth like stomatitis.
- It removes bad odor of the mouth, makes the gum stronger, make teeth stronger.
- It brings softness in the voice and also cures speech related problems, Tonsillitis.

Example

- Ghee and milk it is very useful substance used for the procedure.
- This is done in conditions like mouth ulcer, wounds due to tongue bite or dentition problems, burns.
- It also strengthens the gums, teeth.
- Honey is of sweet quality and has cleansing property which heals the mouth ulcers, helps in dryness of mouth or reduced salivation and enhances taste buds.

Sesame oil

- Sesame oil strengthens the teeth, gives them good luster, strengthens jaws, gums, and enhances taste.
- It imparts good voice; the lips remain moistened eliminating dry or cracked lips.
- The tooth never suffers from caries.
- The teeth will be capable of chewing even the hardest food.

Clove decoction: Clove has a good aroma and it is said to be the best for dental problems.

- When gargling is done with clove decoction, it helps in getting rid of bad odor of mouth.
- It strengthens the teeth and gums, removes toothache or carries.
- Oil pulling is done with various Ayurveda medicated oils like:
- *Ksharambu-* in tonsillitis, excess salivation, reduced taste perception
- *Aragwadadhi Kashaya-* acts as anti-microbic, anti-fungal.

NASAL DROPS

- Nasal drops are the application of medicated liquid, oil, ghee inside the nostrils.
- In Ayurveda it is told that *Kapha* dosha is situated in above neck region and due to *Kapha* there are certain diseases originated like ophthalmic, ENT, neurological disease, psychiatric diseases namely Rhinitis, Polyps, nasal block, Sinusitis etc.

- Nose is said to be the door for head any pathology related to head like headache of various type, vision, and Facial palsy etc. risks can be avoided by instilling nasal drops.
- It also reduces hair fall and enhances growth, stress relief, helps to reduced premature hair graying

Example: plain water (Luke warm), ghee, oil processed with various herbs according to condition of diseases

- Juice of *Bhrngaraja* – Hair fall. Premature graying
- *Anu taila* – hemorrhagic diseases, Hair fall, Alopecia, Epistaxis
- *Trikatu choorna* – Sinusitis, unconsciousness, febrile convulsions
- *Kshira bala taila avartti* – Migraine, dry eye, dry nose, loss of smell, hearing loss, Frozen shoulder, Alzheimer's disease.

COLLYRIUM

- Vision is the most important, so one should protect it with utmost care.
- The eye is most likely to have diseases of *Kapha dosha* so care it.
- Collyrium protects the eyes from disease from imbalance of all *doshas*.
- It is practiced daily by which vision becomes clean, sharp, and beautiful with well grown eye lashes.

Example: Rose water – it having cooling effect helps in Conjunctivitis, foreign body sensation reduced

- *Triphaladi masi* (soot) – corneal opacities, Blephritis, Stye, Chalazion
- *Ilanir kuzhampu* – enhances vision, Conjunctivitis, dry eyes syndrome

EXERCISE

In this fitness maniac era, as observed, people are adopting different ways to remain fit. Some opt healthy, some artificial and sudden weight loss technique whereas some random. Few use harmful pills or drugs; few starve, all these will have adverse effect on long run. People would suffer with organ damage, poor immunity, illness, and reduced strength, and fatigue, mental and physical stress.

There are many healthy ways of exercising which includes

- Walking
- Jogging
- Swimming
- Yoga
- Sports

Ideal time for exercise

- Ideal time is Morning (6 am to 9 am) and evening (4 pm to 6 pm) on empty stomach or after complete digestion of previous meal.
- Here the logic behind the time is body will be fresh, full of stamina and energy, atmosphere will have moderate temperature to minimize excess energy loss.
- As per Ayurveda this time of day *Kapha dosha* is dominant.
- It gives good energy to body and leads to less strain and injuries to muscles, ligaments, and joints.
- If practiced untimely like in noon or night, body suffers lot of energy loss in long run being weak
- This is the time for food intake or rest, where body requires minimal activities.

- Here *Pitha* and *Vata doshas* will be more respectively, so if exercised this part of day causing tiredness, dehydration, muscle cramps, ligament sprain, joint injury, tear in meniscus or other structure.

Suitable environment for exercising
- The environment must be cool, calm, and hygienic, devoid of smoke, extreme temperature, dust, uneven surface.

Season wise
- In season like winter where there is increased body strength the person can use half of body strength.
- In case if he uses more body strength then the *Vata dosha* in body gets disturbed and may cause cramps, sprain or other injuries to bodily structure.
- Thirst will be increased, emaciation, respiratory problems, fatigue physically and mentally, cough, fever, vomiting are commonly seen.
- In other season namely summer, autumn, rainy the exercise is to be performed less.

Breathing technique during exercise
- Slow and study breathing. Deep inhalation and exhalations followed so that there won't be any discomfort while exercising or uneasiness.
- One should never withhold the breath or breath forcefully, if done may cause some breathing problems.

According to one's strength
- People with more body strength like adolescents or middle aged people who have more of *Kapha dosha* should practice it with half of the body strength

- Old age people or children should not indulge in exercise as their body strength is very less or more of *Vata dosha* person should avoid exercising as it causes strain and depletion in body tissue.

Exercise according to body constituency

Person having *Vata dosha*

- Persons should exercise in a mild way, with not much exertion.
- Since the persons will be having comparatively less body strength and rough body parts, weak joints.
- If exerted too much it may lead to injury, cramps, emaciated body, breathing problems.
- Exercises like mild stretching, one which includes least movements and stable movements like
- Yogasana in sitting posture and sleeping posture like *Vrukshasana/ Shashankasana, Vajrasana, Paschimottasana, Pavanamuktasana, Balasana, Shavasana, Pranayama* like *Surya bhedi, Nadi shuddhi* is preferred.

Person having *Pitha dosha*

- One should exercise in mild way without too much exertion.
- Too much Exertion would affect by increased perspiration, rashes on body, prickly heat, giddiness, fatigue, strain on cardiovascular system (high blood pressure).
- Exercises like walking in early morning, swimming,
- *Yogasana* like *Bhujangasana, Shalabhasana, Navasana, Sethubhaddasana*
- *Pranayama* like *Seetali, Sitkari, Chandrabedhi Pranayama.*

Person having *Kapha dosha*

- Here person can use almost ¾th of this body strength for exercising as person will have good body strength and firm joints without much strain or injuries.

- One with *Kapha* dosha will be plumpy so vigorous exercises required to remove excess body fat and shape the body.

Exercises like jogging, cycling
- *Yogasana* like sun salutation, *Trikonasana, Dhanurasana, Shirshasana, Parvathasana, Gomukhasana*, etc.
- *Pranayama* like *Suryabhedhi, Kaphalabhati, Bhramari*.
- Exercise should be practiced daily as to increase the body strength, be efficient in activities, cuts down excess fat from body; body feels light and increases the digestive power. Gives a attractive physique and built and strong body structure.
- A person should exercise until he sweats, body feels light, and muscles are stretched and toned enough, when blood circulation increases, pulse level shoots.
- Contraindicated in those who are diseased because the *dosha* are already imbalanced and body becomes very weak, it will further reduce body strength.
- Exercise should be avoided in small children, old people and in indigestion.

OIL MASSAGE

- Oil massage is application of fat substance/oily substances with certain amount of pressure.
- It is recommended daily.
- It is mainly done to calm down the aggravated *Vata dosha* or to have normal circulation of *Vata dosha* throughout the body.

Classified as per site of body

1. Whole body
2. Single body part
3. Head massage
4. Foot massage

Classified as per modality

1. Massage with hands
2. Massage with foot

Direction of massage

- It is done in direction of hair follicle so that it spreads evenly over the body over chest belly, back.
- Upward massage in regions like calf muscle, upper limbs, neck.
- Circular massage over joints, forehead, jawline.
- It is done in order to ensure correct blood flow, releases stiffness, soreness of muscles.
- It benefits the body as it delays aging process, diminishes the fatigue, improves vision, renders nourishment, god sleep and longevity, improves skin in terms of complexion, tone, elasticity, strong physique.

Ideal time

- In day time almost between 8 am–10 am, before bathing
- It should be done in empty stomach or after complete digestion of previous meal.
- Bowel, bladder and other natural urges are to be fulfilled before massage.

Contraindication

- For those with aggravated *Kapha dosha*, those with poor digestion or indigestion, with fungal, bacterial skin infections.

- Eg: pure coconut oil, seasame oil, gingelly oil
- Oil for people with Vata *dosha*: *Balaashwagandha oil, Kottamchukkadi oil, Mahanarayana taila, Chinchadi oil*
- Oil for people *Pitha dosha*: *Chandanadi oil, Himasagara oil, Ksheerabala oil, Nalpalmaradi oik, Eladi oil, Maduyastyadi oil*
- Oil for people with *Kapha dosha*: *Karpuradi oil, Marichadi oil, Kottamchukkadi oil*

Refer Fig 1.7

POWDER MASSAGE

- Massage to the body is usually done by oil or other substances, but here coarse powder of herbs is used for massage.
- Here the powder is forcefully rubbed over the body in the upward direction (against hair follicles).

Types

1. Dry
2. Oil

Dry powder massage

- Dry, coarse powder is taken for massage. Especially in excess cellulites, excess unctuousness in body, fat under skin in excess, especially for obese.

Unctuous powder massage

- Here powder is made unctuous by adding oil.
- This herbal paste is rubbed over skin.

- Helps to remove dead skin cells, brings about glow to skin, makes the skin soft, increases the skin tone, increases skin complexion.
- It mainly brings down the accumulated *Kapha dosha* in terms of body fat dissolves it away, and provides firmness to the body with excellent clarification of skin.
- Eg: *Triphala* powder for Obesity.
- *Kolakulathadi* powder is best for inflammatory joint disorders.

Refer Fig 1.8

BATH

- Water itself brings life in human. Water being pleasant and cool brings about freshness in human beings.
- Bathing is to be always done with luke warm water, water of room temperature can be used in summer
- It improves the digestion, provided longevity, vitality and vigor, gives strength, energy.
- It keeps the person free from diseases of skin like itching, dirt, fatigue, sweat, tiredness, thirst.
- It removes burning sensation of the body, negative feelings and brings positivity.
- If hot water (medium hot) used for bath for the parts below the neck, then it renders body strength. If hot water used on head then in diminishes vision and hair texture.
- Bathing in cold water in winter and very hot in summer disturbs *Doshas* and causes certain diseases.

- E.g.: in conditions of skin diseases: water boiled with neem.
- Prickly heat, rashes: water boiled with Vetivera roots.
- Soaps containing Aloe Vera, turmeric, sandalwood, *Nalpamara*, basil leaves, coconut oil, jasmine

FOOD

- Food should be taken only after bath as the bath will kindle the digestive fire
- If first eaten then bath, there will arise few digestion problems there must be gap if done so.
- Food should not be eaten before the digestion of prior.
- It should be taken in moderate quantities, not full stomach.
- Quarterly part should be kept empty for proper digestion.

BODY HYGIENE

- Regularly clean or trim hairs, nails, body hairs like moustache/beard or pubic hairs.
- Maintenance of hygiene and cleanliness of orifice like mouth, and excretory is must.
- Take bath daily (twice a day if required), fragrance is used, well dressed, don't wear gaudy attires.
- Always wear jewels, recite sacred hymns and consume divine medicine.
- Sneezing, laughing, yawning should be done by covering the mouth

PROTECTION FROM EXTERNAL ENVIRONMENT

- Carry umbrella while going in sun and rain or while going for long walk.
- Also wear footwear while going out for walk.
- Going out during the night time is to be avoided, if there are unavoidable circumstances it should be aided by helper, or equipped with stick and wearing a cap.

SEASONAL REGIMEN

- STRENGTH OF THE BODY ACCORDING TO THE SEASON   120
- DESCRIPTION OF EACH SEASON (ENVIRONMENTAL STATUS, FOOD AND ACTIVITIES)   120
- SPRING SEASON (*VASANTA*)   122
- SUMMER SEASON (*GREESHMA*)   122
- RAINY SEASON (*VARSHA*)   123
- AUTUMN SEASON (*SARAT*)   125
- EARLY WINTER (*HEMANTA*)   126
- PERIOD OF CLIMATIC CHANGE   126

SEASONAL REGIMEN (*RTHUCHARYA*)

- The variation of multiple factors in each and every season makes considerable changes.
- Thus there is variation in the sleep, food, exercise and other activities according to each season.
- Hence one should accustom to the changes in each season which would endow person a good health.
- This will also help the person to overcome the variations in climate and other changes.
- These are the concepts which help a man to have a systematic life and take him towards a good health physically, mentally and spiritually.

The year is mainly divided into two parts

    1. Solar month – *Uttarayana*

    2. Lunar month – *Dakshinayana*

Seasons		
Extreme winter (*Shishira*)	Jan-Feb	
Spring (*Vasanta*)	March-Apr	Solar month – *Uttarayana*
Summer (*Greeshma*)	May-Jun	
Rainy (*Varsha*)	Jul-Aug	
Autumn (*Sharad*)	Sep-Oct	Lunar month – *Dakshinayana*
Early winter (*Hemanta*)	Nov-Dec	

First three being Solar months (*Uttarayana*) and next three being Lunar months (*Dakshinayana*)

Solar month (*Uttarayana*): It is the half part of the year where the sun has stronger energy than the moon.

- The environment will have sun rays and air having sharp, hot, and dry qualities.
- It thus removes the gentle property of the surroundings.

Lunar month (*Dakshinayana*): It is the next half of the year, during which there be more gentleness.

- The moon is stronger, weakening the sun.
- The environment will be cool, cold.
- There will be clouds, wind, and rain.

STRENGTH OF THE BODY ACCORDING TO THE SEASON

- Maximum strength during the early winter and extreme winter.
- Moderate strength during the spring and autumn.
- Minimal strength during the rainy season and summer.

DESCRIPTION OF EACH SEASON (ENVIRONMENTAL STATUS, FOOD AND ACTIVITIES)

Winter season (*Shishira*)

- The environment will be intensively cold, thus it blocks the external heat flow from the body. It results in increased inner heat i.e. digestive fire.

- Thus the digestion becomes very stronger and hence there will be strong appetite.
- Hence adequate amount of food should be consumed, if not it breaks the tissues.
- In this season night is longer and day shorter. One feels hungry as soon as one wakes up in the morning.

Winter season care		
Food	**Body care**	**Activities**
• Foods with taste like sweet, sour, salty are to be consumed. • Dishes made up of rice, black gram like rice pancake, idly are to be eaten. • Dishes made up of wheat like wheat bread, Pori, wheat pancake, wheat dessert is to be eaten. • Molasses soup. • Sugarcane juice. • Milk and its products like ghee, butter, cottage cheese, and cheese should be consumed in moderate quantity. • Oil should be used in cooking as the body becomes dry. • Oil such as gingelly oil mustard oil, olive oil, coconut oil should be used.	• Application of oil to the scalp and body daily. • Body massage with more pressure is to be done. • Oil like coconut oil, gingelly oil mixed with herbs is used. • Oil namely Pinda taila, *Dhanwantara* oil, *Mahanarayana* oil. • One can also use powders to massage after the oil application with herbs to remove the excess oil. As it removes the excess *Kapha dosha* from the body. • *Triphala* powder, *Kolakulathadi* powder. • Hot water should be used for bath and other toiletry purposes. • Smearing paste of saffron and red sandal wood on the body gives a glow to the skin. • Body should be covered with blankets made up of cotton, silk cloth, and woolen cloths. • Sun bath is advised. One should cover the feet with socks and shoes.	• Exercises are to be done daily which balances the *Vata* and *Kapha doshas*. • It avoids the stiffness of body and cramps of body.

SPRING SEASON (*VASANTA*)

- The *Kapha dosha* is increased due to the predominant cold climate of the previous winter.
- The sun being strong in this season liquefies the *Kapha dosha*.
- Thus weakens the digestive fire and gives rise to various diseases.
- Measures should be taken to pacify the aggravated *Kapha dosha*.
- The increased *Kapha dosha* can be eliminated or pacified depending on the strength of body and many factors.

Spring season care		
Food	**Body care**	**Activities**
• Food having sweet, sour, heavy, unctuous, cold qualities are to be avoided as they increase *Kapha dosha*. • Food should be light which doesn't increase *Kapha dosha*. • Barley, wheat (pan cakes, chapatti, roti, bread). • Meat of arid region (like camel, big horn sheep, kangaroo, buffalo, wild horse, jack rabbit, deer, herons, ostrich, shrimp). • Meat should be directly roasted over fire i.e. grilled or barbeque. • Fermented drinks made up of sugarcane, grape, and honey. • Water boiled with ginger, honey or herbs like *Asana, Musta* can be used for drinking purpose.	• Emesis therapy is best for elimination *Kapha dosha* accumulated in the body. • Powder massages, and foot massage. • Taking bath in hot water later on anointing the body with camphor, sandal, and saffron paste.	• Regular exercises should be done. • Mid-day or noon should be spent sitting on the balcony or veranda, garden, under trees exposing to the breeze. • Day sleep is to be strictly avoided.

SUMMER SEASON (*GREESHMA*)

- In the summer season the sun is very powerful and the climate is humid.
- Thus, it reduces the *doshas* and the body becomes tired.
- So, *Pitha* and *Vata* dosha is imbalanced.

Summer season care

Diet	Body care	Activities
• Food with sweet and mild bitter taste should be taken mainly. • Food with qualities like light, smooth, and cold are to be taken in summer. • Powder of beaten rice with sugar is to be consumed. • White rice cooked with meat soup of wild animals. • Curd, sugar candy, ginger, cumin, salt is churned and mixed with fermented drink like grape wine. • Honey, dates, grapes, dry grapes, sugar with very small amount of camphor should be taken. • Slices of banana and jackfruit stored in brand new clay vessel and kept for fermentation, it turns mildly sour. Then consumed. • Milk of buffalo mixed with sugar is cooled in moonlight. • Taste like salty, spicy, sour must be avoided. • Exercise and exposure to sun is also avoided. • One must not take beverage which is fermented as it has sharp and hot qualities. • If necessary it can be taken in very little quantity diluted with large amount of water.	• Bath should be taken with cold water. • The body should be anointed with paste of sandal. • Thin–smooth, light clothes are to be worn. • Floral garland of cool flowers are to be worn Jewels made up of pearl, coral, sandalwood beads, wearing lotus flower.	• One has to sleep in open garden in night surrounded by trees of palm, pines. • Bed should be surrounded by white cloths which are dipped in cold water. • The walls should be applied with plantain leaf or petals of white water Lilly. • Day sleep or nap is allowed in a cool place. • Before sleeping one should get exposed to the cool moon light, with relaxed mind • One should reduce sexual activities as the body will be weak.

RAINY SEASON (*VARSHA*)

- In the rainy season the sky is surrounded by dark, heavy clouds and wind blowing with droplets of water.
- Therefore when it reaches the earth, it gives out the heat or vapors of acidic nature.

- Thus it aggravates the imbalanced *Vata dosha* (*Pitha* is slightly imbalanced).
- The winter, spring and summer month's leads to weak digestion by reducing the strength of digestive fire.
- Thus it leads to vitiation of all the three *doshas* (mainly *Vata*).
- Diet and activities are followed carefully to increase the digestive fire and bring imbalanced or aggravated *doshas* into normalcy.

Rainy season care		
Diet	**Body care**	**Activities**
• Food which is sour and salty is mixed with adequate amount of smooth substances like ghee, butter. • Eat warm and light food. • Meat soup of arid region (mutton, camel, buffalo) which is seasoned with ghee, mustard, ginger. • Soup of pulses like green gram seasoned with same above. • Old wine, fermented drinks, whey (upper portion of curd) mixed with sochal salt. • Powder of five dry herbs mainly Piper longum, root of Piper longum, piper Brachystachyum, Plumbago zeylanica, and Zingiber officinale boiled in rain water or well water should be drunk warm. • Avoid sweet, spicy, bitter, astringent taste food and heavy foods. • *Karkataka kanji* (rice porridge): a special type of red rice preparation in which other herbs are added and cooked. When eaten in rainy season it pacifies *Vata dosha*, promotes strength and is rejuvenative.	• Water boiled with herbs, should be used for bathing to prevent infections Eg Neem, *Aragwadha*, *Nalpamara*, Vetivera roots. • Steam bath should be taken. • Apply paste of camphor, kumkum with milk and other herbal paste of hot in potency. • Body and cloths should be always fumigated and scented. • Remain in place free from dampness, moisture, cold.	• Remain in warm atmosphere and activities should be minimum. • One should avoid walking without footwear, sleeping during the day, exertion, getting wet in the rain. • Exposure to cold winds, going out during rain or exposure to lightening or thunder are to be strictly avoided.

AUTUMN SEASON (*SARAT*)

- In the autumn season sun is powerful with sharp rays; it aggravates the accumulated *Pitha dosha* in the body. Thus the body gets extremely warm causing various diseases.
- In rainy season the atmosphere is cold.

Autumn season care		
Diet	Body care	Activities
• Measures should be taken to pacify the *Pitha dosha*. • Ghee is the best to pacify *Pitha dosha*. • Food having taste of bitter, sweet, astringent is best to pacify *Pitha dosha*. • Light food like rice, green gram, Indian gooseberry, sugar, milk, snake gourd, honey. • Wild meat (mutton, sheep, buffalo, and camel) should be taken in moderate quantity. • Heavy food, alkaline substances (vinegar, baked food), gingelly or sesame oil are to be avoided.	• Oil massage and steam bath are the best in the season. • Body is anointed by paste of sandal wood, camphor. • Chains made of pearl should be worn. Body should be exposed to the moon light. • Decoction of herbs with milk is poured all over the body. • Purgation is the best measure to eliminate excess vitiated • *Pitha dosha*. • With *Tiktaka ghritha*, • *Mahatiktaka ghritha*. • *Shirodhara* should be done with milk and herbs like *Amalaki, Jatamamsi*. • Bath with moderately warm water. • Bloodletting is other therapy to pacify the *Pitha dosha*.	• Moderate body exercises like *Yoga*, crunches, and pushups can be done. • Exposure to chimney fire or bon fire. • Things to be avoided 1. Exposure to fog 2. Day sleep

Water

- The water heated with sun rays in the day and cooled by exposing to external atmosphere at night is the best for drinking in this season.
- It becomes capable of pacifying the three *doshas* and acts like elixir.

EARLY WINTER (*HEMANTA*)

- Atmospheric condition is same as that of the late winter or extreme winter, but with low intensity.
- The regimen followed here is similar to that of extreme winter.

Recommendation of taste according to the season

Taste of food to be eaten	Season
Sweet, sour, salty	early winter, extreme winter, rainy season
Bitter, astringent, spicy	spring season
Sweet	summer season
Sweet, bitter, astringent	autumn season

PERIOD OF CLIMATIC CHANGE

- The last seven days of a season and first seven days of next season is considered as period of climatic change.
- This particular period is difficult for the body to adjust to the changes as a reason; the body gets sensitive and weaker.
- The three *doshas* gets disturbed, hence proper measures should be taken.
- In these 14 days, previous seasonal regimen should be gradually reduced and the next season regimens are to be followed.
- If the regimen is suddenly changed, it will be difficult for the body to adjust.
- Slow and gradual change should be brought in the regimen.

CLASSIFICATION OF TREATMENT ACCORDING TO AYURVEDA

- TWO FOLDS OF TREATMENTS 129
- THREE FOLDS OF TREATMENTS 129

CLASSIFICATION OF TREATMENT ACCORDING TO AYURVEDA

TWO FOLDS OF TREATMENTS

- Treatment in Ayurveda is mainly classified as *Antarparimarjana* and *Bahirparimarjana*.
- *Antarparimarjana* means taking medicines internally.
- The medicines are given in the form of decoctions, tablets, powder etc.
- It is advised in almost all the stages of disease.
- *Bahirparimarjana* means external treatments.
- It is advised in conditions of severe pain, swelling, injury, skin rashes.
- It is also mainly advised in low back pain, knee joint pain, loss of sleep etc.
- A few examples are in pain, swelling: paste of *Nagaradi choorna, Kottamchukkadi choorna.*
- In skin rashes: paste of *Dashanga choorna, Shatadhouta ghrita.*

THREE FOLDS OF TREATMENTS

- The three folds of treatments are *Daivavyapasraya, Yuktivyapasraya* and *Satvavajaya.*

- *Daivavyapasraya* means divine therapy.
- A few of the diseases are not curable by medicines as the origin of the disease is found to be by previous birth misdeeds.
- Such diseases are managed by *Homa* therapy, chanting *Mantra*, wearing specific germ stones according to one's birth stones.
- Charity, fasting are the modes.
- *Yuktivyapasraya* means logical usage of treatments according to the disease.
- It may be in the form of external or internal treatments.
- *Satvavajaya* means psychotherapy.
- Diseases which are mainly psychological in nature are treated mainly by a positive counseling rather than just medicines.
- In the present day most of the diseases has mind involved.
- Calming the person, giving assurance, moral support, encouraging the patients to participate in pleasureful activities will help him.
- The above approaches will make one's mind stable and strong.

DETOXIFICATION THERAPIES

- *SNEHAPANA* (GHEE THERAPY)   134
- *SWEDANA* (SWEATING/SUDATION THERAPY)   134
- *VAMANA* (VOMITING OR EMESIS THERAPY)   135
- *VIRECHANA* (PURGATION THERAPY, LOOSE STOOLS)   137
- *VASTHI* (ENEMA)   140
- *RAKTAMOKSHANA* (BLOODLETTING)   140
- *RASAYANA* (REJUVENATION THERAPY)   141

DETOXIFICATION THERAPIES (PANCHAKARMA)

When a cloth is full of dirt, it cannot be used unless and until it is cleaned. Similarly when the body is full of toxins or dirt, it causes diseases.

There is a major need for the body to be cleansed and the toxins should be eliminated.

Detoxification therapies are to be done under utmost care with a supervision of skillful or experienced physician.

During this period there will be strict diet and activity restrictions, since therapies are strong for the body.

The five Detoxification or Purification therapies are

1. Emesis/Vomiting
2. Purgation
3. Nasal drops
4. Decoction enema
5. Oil enema

- Difference of opinion

1. Emesis
2. Purgation/Loose bowels
3. Nasal drops
4. Enema
5. Blood letting

SNEHAPANA (GHEE THERAPY)

§ Ghee is the best fat of the (Ghee, oil, muscle fat, bone marrow) four fats.

§ Ghee has the property to mix with herbs, and attain the properties of herbs mixed with it. Ghee has the smooth and sticky quality which can reach the minutest parts and toxins gets sticked to it.

§ Ghee with combination of various herbs is used for different conditions or diseases.
- *Indukantha Ghrita*: Immunity, Digestive disorders, Arthrittis
- *Tiktaka Ghrita*: Skin disorders.
- *Kalyanaka Ghrita*: Mental wellbeing and Male infertility.
- *Brahmi Ghrita*: Psychological disorders.
- *Guggulutikta Ghrita*: Diabetes, high cholesterol level, Obesity.
- *Phala Sarpis*: Female infertility.

§ The ghee is initially given in test dose or small quantity.

§ Depending upon the person's digestive capacity and strength, the dose of the ghee is gradually increased.

§ Ghee has property of crossing blood brain barrier. This means that Ghee can penetrate into the deeper tissues, bring the accumulated toxins or metabolic wastes with it.

Refer Fig 1.9

SWEDANA (SWEATING/SUDATION THERAPY)

- Sweating is the therapy where heat is subjected to the body and the aggravated toxins (by Ghee therapy) is liquefied.

- The liquefied toxins move towards the stomach from the different parts of body.
- Later the patient is given fat rich food on the previous day of Vomiting therapy/Purgation therapy.
- This will stimulate the toxins which have settled in the stomach and thus the patient is made ready for Vomiting therapy/Purgation therapy.
- The stronger form of sweating therapy is *Bashpa sweda*, where whole body is subjected to steam chamber except the head and neck.
- The mild form of Sweating therapy is widely used as general treatment.
- Forms of mild Sweating therapy are;
    1. Pouch massage with lemon, or herbs or powder.
    2. Exposure to steam through tube connected to pressure cooker (Localized).
    3. Pouring of herbal liquid all over the body.
    4. Pouring of Ayurveda vinegar all over the body.
- Exposure to sunlight, covering heavy blankets, remaining in completely closed room without ventilation are other Sweating therapies without fire.

VAMANA (VOMITING OR EMESIS THERAPY)

- Vomiting is the one among the Detoxification therapies where the aggravated toxins are removed or eliminated from upper route i.e. mouth.
- This procedure is mainly done to pacify the *Kapha dosha*.
- The therapy is done after two major processes namely Ghee therapy and Sweating therapy

Pre-vomiting diet

The pre vomiting diet consists of food which triggers the *Kapha dosha*.

- Breakfast: Black gram pan cake with coconut sauce and 1 glass of milk.
- Lunch: Curd rice and 1 glass of milk.
- Dinner: Sweet milk porridge, Semolina desert.

Time of procedure

- The person/patient should fresh up and come to the treatment room.
- One should Pray God; accept the medicine wholeheartedly so that the medicine works its best.
- Vomiting or emesis should be done early morning around 5 am.

Main medicines used:

- Liquorice: Glychrizza glabra powder.
- Emetic nut: Randia dumetorum
- Sweet flag: Acorus calamus
- Grapes: Vitis vinifera decoction
- Milk
- Salt water

The person should vomit continuously until the contents in the stomach are emptied.

- Incase improper vomiting occurs, it may cause indigestion and aggravates skin problems.
- Duration: 45–60 min.
- Later the patient is advised to take rest.
- After 3 hours after vomiting, the patient is advised to take breakfast.

Diet after vomiting therapy

- Day of vomiting
- Breakfast: Rice water
- Lunch: rice porridge (without milk)
- Dinner: kichadi

Indications

In cases like,

- Depression, Psoriasis, Eczema, Hypothyroidism, Epilepsy, Attention deficit syndrome, Food poisoning, Female infertility.
- Not advised conditions:
- Hypertension, Heart problems, Tumor, Pneumonia, Tuberculosis, Bleeding conditions, Old age, Pregnancy, Children.

VIRECHANA (PURGATION THERAPY, LOOSE STOOLS)

- Purgation means taking medicines orally which removes the toxins through downward route i.e. anus.
- This therapy is mainly beneficial for pacifying the *Pitha dosha*.
- This procedure is started with Ghee therapy that lasts for 3–7 days.
- Later 2 days of oil massage and steam bath.
- Pre purgation diet
- Breakfast: lemon rice with pickle
- Lunch: tomato rice with lemon juice
- Dinner: lemon rice with pickle and lemon juice
- Time: around 9 am.

- After morning bath in empty stomach.
- One should Pray God; accept the medicine wholeheartedly so that the medicine works its best.

Medicine used is

- *Triphala* decoction (strong purgation): skin disorders, Obesity.
- *Trivrith lehya*: pacifies skin disorders, *Pitha dosha*.
- Castor oil with milk or warm water: pacifies *Vata dosha* arthritis, low back pain, constipation.
- Avipathi choorna: mild and safest to take, pacifies mainly *Pitha dosha*.
- The patient is advised to drink warm water in between, which stimulates the intestine and helps in complete elimination of toxins.
- The patient may have loose stools for about 10–30 times.
- If it crosses 30 or if person feels giddiness or weakness, it should be stopped by taking cold water or cold lemon water.

Food after purgation therapy

- The time when purgation slows down or patient feels very tired rice water should be given.
- The next day morning rice porridge (without milk) should be given.
- According to the person's appetite and number of loose stools, the food should be decided.
- Kichadi is a special dish that can be given after the Detoxification therapy as it is light and easy digestible.

Indications

In cases like,

- Liver cirrhosis, Jaundice, Constipation, Urinary incontinence, Skin disorders like Eczema, Psoriasis, Dermatitis, Acne vulgaris, Bronchial asthma, Vitiligo, Urticuria, Fatty liver, Gouty arthritis.

Not advised in conditions like,

- Bleeding piles, Rectal prolapse, Intestinal obstruction, Dehydration, and Irritable bowel disease, Ulcers in stomach or intestines, Debility, old age, pregnant, children.

Nasya (Nasal drops)

- Nose is the gateway for head.
- *Nasya* is the administration of drops into the nose. (Oil is used commonly, fine herbal powder/fresh extracted herbal juice)

Before putting the nasal drops,

The face, neck and back are massaged with warm oil and steam is given to the face.

Time: 8–9 am

Common oils: *Anu taila, Shadbindu taila*

The patient is advised to lie down with head lower than the level of body.

- Patient is advised to inhale deeply.
- Patient is then advised to completely spit out the drops that reach the throat.

Indications: Sinusitis, Migraine, Cervical spondylosis, Insomnia.

Refer Fig 2.0

VASTHI (ENEMA)

- *Vasthi* means pushing the oil or herbal liquid into the anus.
- The treatment that reaches up to the level of the urinary bladder is known as *Vasthi*.
- This procedure also reaches up to the level of intestine, which is the site of *Vata* dosha.
- Hence it is the best treatment for *Vata dosha*.
- Types: Oil enema: to be done after lunch around 2.30 pm.
- Herbal decoction enema: around 4.30 pm.

Indications: Sciatica, Multiple sclerosis, Parkinsonism, Infertility, Irritable bowel syndrome, Rheumatoid arthritis, Gouty arthritis, Ankolysis spondylosis.

Refer Fig 2.1

RAKTAMOKSHANA (BLOODLETTING)

Raktamokshana is the treatment where impure blood is removed from body with the help of leeches or other instruments.

Time: after lunch.

Indications: Varicosity, Raynaud's phenomenon, Acne vulgaris.

Refer Fig 2.2

How often one should do the Detoxification therapies?

One should do either of Detoxification therapies according to one's condition at least once in a year.

This is essential because of one's bad food habits and lifestyle in the present life.

Age limit for Detoxification therapies: above the age of 18 years up to the age of 70 years.

RASAYANA (REJUVENATION THERAPY)

- The person after undergoing the Detoxification therapies must undergo Rejuvenation therapies.
- The medicines absorbs into the body easily after Purification therapies.
- The below given is the best practical way of usage of different rejuvenative medicines at ones respective age.

Age	Rejuvenative medicine
1 month to 14 years	Gold drops with different herbs (*Swarna prashana*)
18–40 years	*Chyavanaprasha, Brahma rasayana, Narasimha rasayana*
40–60 years	Women: *Shatavari lehya*
	Men: *Aswagandha rasayana*

- Aging is gradual phenomenon.
- As a man passes different ages he is bound to have physiological as well as psychological changes in the body.
- The *Rasayana* will help in maintaining aging and prevent early degeneration.

EXTERNAL TREATMENTS IN AYURVEDA

- SHIRO DHARA — 145
- SHIRO VASTI — 145
- TALA PODICHIL — 146
- KARNA POORANA — 146
- NETRA TARPANA — 146
- GRIVA VASTI — 147
- KATI VASTI — 147
- JANU VASTI — 148
- NARANGA KIZHI — 148
- ELA KIZHI — 148
- PODI KIZHI — 149
- NJAVARA KIZHI — 149
- PIZHICHIL — 150
- SARVANGA KASHAYA DHARA/KSHEERA DHARA — 150

EXTERNAL TREATMENTS IN AYURVEDA

SHIRO DHARA

- *Shiro* means head and *dhara* means pouring.
- Pouring of oil/medicated milk/medicated butter milk in the forehead in rhythmic oscillations is called *Shiro dhara*.
- The medicated liquid or oil is poured on forehead through *dhara* pot which is hanged over a stand.
- The pouring should be continuous, from one end of forehead to other.

Duration: 30–45 min

Benefits: Effective for Stress, Anxiety, Mania, loss of sleep and other disturbances, Psoriasis and other skin problems, Hypothyroidism, Migraine, Hair fall, Dandruff, Hypertension.

Refer Fig 2.3

SHIRO VASTI

- *Shiro vasti* means retaining oil on the head.
- A vertical cap made of leather is placed over the head, which is fixed firmly.
- Warm oil around 250–500 ml is retained over the head.
- The oil should always remain warm.

Duration: 20–30 min

Note: hairs should be trimmed/cut short to have best results.

Benefits: Effective in Parkinsonism, Alzheimer's disease, Stroke, Facial palsy, Sleep disturbances.

Refer Fig 2.4

TALA PODICHIL

- *Tala podichil* means applying herbal paste on the head, and wrapping it with banana leaf.

Duration: 30–40 min

Benefits: Effective in Anxiety, Stress, Insomnia, Premature greying of hairs, Hair fall.

KARNA POORANA

- *Karna poorana* means bathing the ear in warm oil.

Duration: 15–20 min

Benefits: Effective in hearing disorders, Tinnitus, ear ache, excess ear wax, dryness in the ear canal and itching.

NETRA TARPANA

- *Netra Tarpana* means retention of medicated ghee over the eyes.
- Eyes are surrounded by circular shaped wheat dough with warm ghee filled in it.

- Patient is advised to blink eyes repeatedly while the ghee is retained over the eyes.

Duration: 5–15 min

Benefits: Effective in increasing clarity of vision, correcting refractive errors, eye strain.

Refer Fig 2.5

GRIVA VASTI

- *Griva vasti* means retaining of warm oil over the neck.
- A compartment is made out of wheat dough over the nape of neck; inside it the medicated oil is retained.

Duration: 30–45 min

Benefits: Effective in Cervical spondylosis, Cervical sprain, Tension headache, Migraine.

KATI VASTI

- *Kati vasti* means retaining of warm oil over the lower back (lumbar-sacral region)
- A compartment is made out of wheat dough over the lower back; inside it the medicated oil is retained.

Duration: 30–45 min

Benefits: Effective for Sciatica, IVDP, Lumbar stenosis.

Refer Fig 2.6

JANU VASTI

- *Janu vasti* means retaining of warm oil over the knee joint.
- A compartment is made out of wheat dough over the knee joint; inside it the medicated oil is retained.

Duration: 30–45 min

Benefits: Osteo arthritis, Osteo porosis, Meniscal tear.

NARANGA KIZHI

- *Naranga kizhi* means the pouch massage with lemon in it.
- The massage is done is rhythmic manner over the affected part or whole body with lemon, turmeric, rock salt, garlic inside it.
- The pouch should always remain warm throughout the massage.

Duration: 30–45 min

Benefits: Effective in Low back pain, Sciatica, Neck pain or sprain, Rheumatoid arthritis.

ELA KIZHI

- *Ela kizhi* means the pouch massage with herbal leaves in it.
- The massage is done is rhythmic manner over the affected part or whole body with leaves of *Nirgundi, Arka, Eranda* etc along with turmeric, rock salt, garlic inside it.
- The pouch should always remain warm throughout the massage.

Duration: 30–45 min

Benefits: Effective in Cervical Spondylosis, Osteo arthritis, Rheumatoid arthritis, Frozen shoulder, Tennis elbow.

Refer Fig 2.7

PODI KIZHI

- *Podi kizhi* means the pouch massage with powder in it.
- The massage is done is rhythmic manner over the affected part or whole body with mixture of different herbal dry powders inside it.
- The pouch should always remain warm throughout the massage.

Duration: 30–45 min

Benefits: Effective in Osteo arthritis, Obesity, Diabetic neuropathy, Rheumatoid arthritis.

NJAVARA KIZHI

- *Njavra kizhi* means the pouch massage with cooked red rice (*Njavara*) in it.
- The massage is done is rhythmic manner over the affected part or whole and should be heated frequently as it gets cold soon.

Duration: 30–40 min

Benefits: It is nourishing and improves the skin tone, strengthens the muscles, nervous system and rejuvenates the body. Effective in Muscular degeneration, Debility, Stroke.

Refer Fig 2.8

PIZHICHIL

- *Pizhichil* means pouring warm medicated oil all over the body.
- The warm medicated oil is poured in the height of 2–3 inches.

Duration: 30–45 min

Benefits: Effective in Chronic fatigue syndrome, Loss of weight, Neurological disorders like Motor Neuron disease, Multiple Sclerosis, Parkinsonism.

Refer Fig 2.9

SARVANGA KASHAYA DHARA/KSHEERA DHARA

- *Sarvanga kashaya dhara/Ksheera dhara* means pouring of herbal decoction/herbal decoction of milk all over the body.
- Warm decoction is poured over the affected parts or all over the body with the height of 2–3 inches.

Duration: 30–45 min

Benefits: Effective in improving blood circulation, reduces joint pain and inflammation.

Effective in Skin disorders, Degenerative joint disease and joint stiffness.

Refer Fig 3.0

OLD AGE RELATED DISEASES

- RHEUMATOID ARTHRITIS 153
- DEMENTIA 155
- SENILITY 156
- ANXIETY 158
- URINARY INCONTINENCE 159

OLD AGE RELATED DISEASES

RHEUMATOID ARTHRITIS

- Rheumatoid arthritis is the most common affected disease in the elderly. It is also an auto immune disease.
- It is commonly seen after the age of 50 years.
- But now days it is common even in the age of 30 years due to sedentary lifestyle.

Symptoms
- Pain in the small joints mainly finger joints and toes etc.
- Early morning stiffness in the body.
- Difficulty in all the movements of the affected joints.
- Swelling in the affected joints.
- Various deformities in the finger joints like swan neck deformity, z neck deformity etc.

Ayurveda approach
- In this disease, the dry, cold nature of *Vata dosha* is vitiated due to the formation of undigested matter.
- The reason for the formation of the undigested matter is due to the bad food habits and eating heavy food, even during low digestive fire.

- Activities like exposure to the cold suddenly soon after to exposure to hot environment.
- So one has to pacify the *Vata dosha* by hot potency, and digest the undigested matter.
- One has to throw it out from body through carminative and digestive food and medicines.
- Ginger is the best remedy for Rheumatoid arthritis as it digests the undigested particles.
- Dry treatments are adopted in this disease like pouch massage with herbs, powder and sand.
- One can also do stretching exercise as well as swimming, which improves flexibility and joint movements.
- Castor oil is one of the best remedy for Arthritis. Castor oil around 1 tsp. can be taken with hot water night.
- Bandages with paste around the finger joints is another good remedy.
- One should take warm food, properly cooked food.
- It is better to take salads in lunch time and steamed vegetables in the night.
- One should take ginger water, add ginger garlic more in food preparation.
- One should take more porridge preparations like rice porridge, or milk into it.

Ayurveda medicines like
- *Maharasnadi Kashaya*
- *Dhanwantara Kashaya*
- *Yogaraja guggulu*

- *Simhanada guggulu*
- *Kashaya* should be taken 20 ml before breakfast and dinner.
- All the medicines helps to correct metabolism, reduce the pain, inflammation, swelling, further degeneration.
- Guggulus in the dose of 2 tablets after breakfast and dinner.
- Oils for application (Oil should be avoided in the starting stage of disease, it may increase inflammation)
- *Kottamchukadi taila*
- *Mahanarayana taila*
- Creams, pastes like;
- *Nagaradi choorna* (powder), *Shallaki* ointment (best pain reliever, anti-inflammatory property)

Refer Fig 3.1

DEMENTIA

- Loss of memory is known as Dementia.
- In this condition a person forgets even recent things.
- There will be lack of recollection, concentration, absent mindness.
- It is mainly related to functions of the brain and due to degeneration.

Symptoms

- Inability to recollect even recent things.
- Forgetting important events like one's own birthday, forgetting to add salt or sugar while preparing food.
- Forgetfulness is the main symptom.

Ayurveda approach

- One has to take food which regenerates the brain tissues.
- Rejuvenation form of treatment is the best for Dementia.
- One should take milk and ghee in the diet as it helps in tissue regeneration.
- Vegetables like pumpkin, ash gourd, spinach, amaranth etc.
- Fruits like grapes, pomegranate, and banana.
- Take small fishes like mackerel, tuna; nuts like cashew nuts and hazelnuts.
- One can grind *Mandokaparni* leaves with coconut and eat as food.
- One should do more mind games, try to sit and recollect.

Ayurveda medicines like

- *Brahmi* tablets: 2 tablets twice a day after food.
- *Shankhapushpi* syrup: 10 ml twice a day after food.
- *Kalyanaka Ghrita:* 5 ml empty stomach.
- *Brahmi Ghrita:* 5 ml empty stomach.
- *Kushmanda rasyana:* 5 gm after breakfast.
- *Saraswatharishta:* 30 ml twice a day after food.
- All the medicines helps to increase the memory, intelligence, concentration.

SENILITY

- Senility is a condition due to ageing.

Symptoms

- Weakness all over the body.
- Feeling tired throughout the day.

- Loss of memory
- Loss of hearing, defective vision.
- Lack of sexual vigor and excitement.
- Multiple joint pain.

Ayurveda approach

- Main line of treatment is to strengthen the nerves, body, joint, mind.
- Food and treatment should be regenerative, strengthening and rejuvinative.
- Rice, wheat, ragi should be consumed as it helps in tissue building.
- Vegetables like ash gourd, spinach, carrot, beetroot and broccoli are the best.
- Fruits like grapes, pomegranate, avocadoes, and berries are good.
- One has also take milk, yogurt, soya, tofu and calcium rich products.
- Egg, mutton soup are the best source for calcium which helps in reducing the bone degeneration.

Ayurveda medicines like

Ashwagandha choorna: 2 tsp. with warm milk or hot water after bed time. (A very good nerve tonic, strengthens the body, mind, an powerful antioxidant, promotes sexual vigour, testosterone hormone).

Kapikachu choorna: 2 tspn. with warm milk or hot water after bed time.
- It helps to strengthen the neurons, nervous system, as well as increase sexual potency.

Brahma rasayana: 2 tsp. with warm milk after breakfast.
- A very good medicine for the neurons which supply the brain as well as oxygenation of the cells.

External application:

- *Bala ashwagandhadi taila, ksira bala taila, Maha masha taila on the body.*: strengthens the body as well as nourishes the muscles and cells.

ANXIETY

Feeling of fear about life.

Symptoms

- Feeling of lack of confidence in life.
- Feeling restless doing activities.
- Worrying and hurrying over things e.g.: panicking partner on previous night of travelling next day.
- Feeling of loneliness in life.

Ayurveda approach

- Social interaction among the family.
- One should involve in daily conversation among the family members.
- One should involve in various activities like gardening, cleaning rooms, walking, attending various functions like social gatherings like Christmas, marriage, birthday.
- Travelling and exploring places like India.
- Visiting places of worship daily like temples, churches, and mosques. And daily offering prayer to the God.
- Listening to melodious music.

Jatamamsi choorna: 2 tspn. of powder with warm water twice a day after dinner

- It is very effective for anxiety, stress and a very good nerve relaxant.

Tagara capsules: 2 capsules at bed time.

- Acts as anti-anxiety, anti-stress.

Ashwagandharishta: 30 ml after breakfast and dinner

- It is a nerve tonic, nerve strengthening, acts as anti-anxiety.

External application:

- *Jatamamsi* paste over vertex: calms the mind, anxiolytic, promotes sleep.
- *Kachuradi choorna*: same action above
- *Ksira bala taila*: strengthens the brain, sensory organs, calms the mind.
- *Himasagara taila*: cools the brain, removes tension of brain, mind.

URINARY INCONTINENCE

Symptoms

- Increased frequency of urine is the main symptom.
- Burning sensation in the urine.
- Pain while micturition.
- Discoloration of urine.
- Fever

Ayurveda approach

- Avoid dairy products.
- Avoid tuna, prawns, shell fish.
- Avoid ice-creams, egg.
- One should include more;
- *Sarasparila* water
- Lemon water
- Ginger water
- Coriander
- Barley water

Ayurveda medicines like

Chandraprabha vati: 2 tablets after breakfast and dinner

- It helps to regulate the functions of the urinary system and reduces urinary infection.

Shiva gutika, Gokshura guggulu: 2 tablets after breakfast and dinner

- It helps in urinary infection.

Gomutra: 10 ml after breakfast.

MIDDLE AGE REALTED DISEASES

- DIABETES MELLITUS 163
- HYPERCHOLESTERAMIA 165
- HYPOTHYROIDISM 166
- PCOS 168
- MENOPAUSAL SYNDROME 170
- HYPERTENSION 172
- LOW BACK ACHE 173
- OBESITY 174
- DEPRESSION 176

MIDDLE AGE RELATED DISEASES

DIABETES MELLITUS

- Diabetes mellitus is a sedentary lifestyle disease and also caused by unhealthy food habits.

Symptoms

- Increased frequency of urine.
- Increased thirst.
- Increased hunger
- Numbness or pain in legs.
- Dark yellow color urine.
- Tiredness during the day.

Ayurveda approach

- One should have a regular diet and healthy lifestyle.
- One should do increased movements to all parts of the body like brisk walking, swimming Yoga like *Shashankasana* (rabbit pose), *Paschimotasana* (seated forward bend), *Halasana* (plough pose), *Dhanurasana* (bow pose).
- Pranayama like *Anuloma viloma, Kapala bathi* and *Bhramari*.

- Frequent, small portions of meals.
- One should sleep correct time or irregular sleep patterns increases the tiredness in the body.

Don'ts
- Avoid too much rice, dairy products.
- Avoid lazy postures like laying on bed whole time or lying on chair.
- Avoid untimely, heavy meals.

Ayurveda medicines like

Nishamalaki choorna: 2 teaspoon with glass of warm water after lunch and dinner.
- It maintains the blood glucose levels, provides anti-oxidants which relieves tiredness.

Chandraprabha vati: 2 tablets after breakfast and lunch.
- It maintains the flow of urine, normalizes the blood glucose levels, and provides rejuvenation to the cells.

Triphala choorna: 2 teaspoon with glass of warm water after lunch and dinner
- A very good antioxidant, corrects the blood glucose levels, prevents Diabetic complications like Diabetes retinopathy.

Food
- One should add more fenugreek powder, curcuma, cinnamon, ginger, curry leaves in the diet.
- Avoid all fruits except guava, green apples, Indian gooseberry.
- Take more bitter gourd, snake gourd, cucumber, salads, green leafy vegetables like spinach etc.

HYPERCHOLESTERAMIA

The condition is mainly a sign and not symptom.

Symptoms

- Increased levels of total cholesterol.
- Increased levels of triglycerides (TG).
- Increased levels of low density lipoproteins (LDL: Bad cholesterol).
- Increased levels of very low density lipoproteins (VLDL).
- Decreased levels of high density lipoproteins (HDL).

Ayurveda approach

- Main importance should be given to maintain the blood cholesterol levels by diet and exercise.

Food

Do's

- Green leafy vegetables, curry leaves; add more fenugreek seeds, garlic, ginger, turmeric into diet.
- Take nuts like peanuts, groundnuts, walnuts.
- Take cinnamon powder 2 tspn. with honey 1 tsp.
- One can take green tea, butter milk, Garcinia indica fruit (Cocoum), jamun fruit.
- One can take empty stomach: fenugreek seeds.
- One should take white meat like breast of chicken; small fishes like sardine, mackerel, tuna.

Don'ts

- Avoid red meat
- Reduce intake of dairy products especially cottage cheese, ghee.
- Avoid pastries, ice creams
- Avoid sitting idle and day sleep.

Ayurveda medicines like

Varunadi Kashaya: 20 ml with glass of lukewarm water before breakfast and dinner.

Navaka guugulu: 2 tablets after breakfast and dinner.

Triphala choorna: 2 tsp. with warm water bed time

Varasanadi kashaya: 20 ml with glass of lukewarm water before breakfast and dinner.

Mode of action of the medicines: depletes the body fat, maintains the blood cholesterol, and corrects the fat metabolism.

HYPOTHYROIDISM

- Hypothyroidism is the disorder related to thyroid gland where the thyroid becomes inactive.
- As a result it causes harmful effects over the body and hampers the metabolism.
- TSH levels are increased due to under active thyroid.

Symptoms

- Major symptoms are weight gain, central obesity.
- Lethargy or feeling cold.

- Hair loss or dry hairs.
- Skin changes like dry skin, increased pigmentation.
- High cholesterol.
- Irregular menstruation.
- Mood disorders like irritability, Depression

Ayurveda approach

- Treating improper fat metabolism and elevated TSH levels.
- Diet and lifestyle should be corrected.

Do's

- Food with more of bitter, astringent taste should be taken.
- E.g.: Snake gourd, Ivory gourd, Bitter gourd, Lettuce, Okra, Capsicum, Long beans, Carrots, Beetroots.
- Spices should be used in moderate quantity like Cinnamon, Fennel seeds, Fenugreek seeds, Black Pepper.
- Fruits like Papaya, Pomegranates, Apple, Oranges, Lemon, Berries, Avocado, and Kiwi
- Nuts like Almonds, Figs, Raisins, Walnut should be used.

Don'ts

- Avoid food with Sweet and Salty taste.
- E.g.: Milk and Milk products esp. Yogurt, Desserts, Aerated drinks, baked food, fried food and processed food.
- Meat of Pork, Mutton, Beef are to be strictly avoided.

Ayurveda medicines like

Hamsapathiyadi kashaya: 10 ml with warm water empty stomach and before food in the evening.

- It helps in balancing the TSH levels.

Kanchanara guggulu: 2 tablets after breakfast and dinner.

- It corrects the fat metabolism

N.A.C + Triphala choorna: mixed together- ½ tsp. with 200 ml water is boiled and reduced to 100 ml and decoction is prepared.

- 100 ml decoction should be taken in empty stomach in the morning and before dinner.
- It helps to improve the sluggish metabolism thus balances the TSH levels.
- Along with medicine and diet, physical activities like yoga and exercises are equally important.

PCOS

- Polycystic ovarian syndrome is a complex form of disorder that affects females of teenage or middle age.
- It is a hormonal imbalance which causes ovaries to enlarge and form multiple cysts around it.

Symptoms

- Irregular menstrual cycle.
- Increased or decreased menstrual bleeding, painful menstruation.
- Skin changes like Acne, Pigmentation, and Facial Hair growth.
- Changes in metabolism leading to puffiness in body, Weight gain and Constipation.
- Hair fall, dry hairs, Dandruff.
- Mood swings like Anxiety/Depression.
- Infertility as it hampers ovulation.

Ayurveda approach

- Balancing the hormones
- Correcting the menstrual irregularity
- Diet, sleep patterns and lifestyle should be corrected

Do's

- Eat high fiber food like Beans, Spinach, Amaranth, Broccoli, Beetroot, Ridge gourd.
- Fruits like Papaya, Pears, Plums, Peach, Strawberries, Grapes, Apples
- Spices like Turmeric, Cumin, Fenugreek, Asafetida, Cinnamon, Black Pepper, Black Sesame.
- Nuts and dry fruits like Almonds, Figs, Apricot, Walnut, Hazelnuts
- Fish like Salmon, Sardines, Tuna, and Silverfish.
- Physical Activities like Yoga, Cycling, Jogging, and Walking.

Don'ts

- Avoid dairy products like cheese, Yogurt.
- Meat like red meats (Pork, Beef, Mutton)
- Sugary drinks, Aerated drinks, Junk, Baked, Frozen, Processed food are to be strictly avoided.

Ayurveda medicines like

Saptasaram Kashayam: 20 ml with glass of lukewarm water before breakfast and dinner

- It reduces menstrual discomfort, and regulates the flow.

Kulathadi kashyam: 20 ml with glass of lukewarm water before breakfast and dinner

- It is used in Amenorrhea or less menstrual bleeding

Kumaryasava: 30 ml after breakfast and dinner.

- It is used in Amenorrhea or less menstrual bleeding

Ashokarista: 30 ml after breakfast and dinner.

- It acts upon the uterus; it is helpful to control excess menstrual flow and reduces menstrual pain and uterine tonic.

Hingu vachadi Tablet: 2 tablets after breakfast and dinner

- It is used in Amenorrhea or less menstrual bleeding

Rajapravarthini vati: 2 tablets after breakfast and dinner

- It corrects Amenorrhea or less menstrual bleeding

Pushyanuga choorna: ½ tsp. with warm water morning and evening before food

- It is helpful to control excess menstrual flow and regulates cycles.

MENOPAUSAL SYNDROME

- Women suffer from Menopausal syndrome between the ages of 40–50 years, where hormonal variation affects a lot.

Symptoms
- Body cramps
- Hot flushes
- Mood swings
- Weight gain
- Cellulite formation
- High blood pressure or low blood pressure

- Hair fall
- Disturbance in vision
- Skin changes like Hyperpigmentation, tanning or dullness in complexion, dryness in body
- Irregular menstruation
- Lack of sexual interest

Ayurveda approach

- The main aim is to maintain the hormone levels which are the main cause for all the symptoms.
- One should take more fruits such as grapes, pomegranates, water melon, banana, melon, figs, and berries.
- Avoid dry foods such as nuts, popcorns.
- Reduce salt intake.
- Coconut water helps in relieving the menstrual cramps.

Ayurveda medicines like

Shatavari gulam: 2 tsp. with warm milk after breakfast.
- It helps to reduce the menstrual cramps, maintain the Estrogen hormone levels, helps in mood swings.

Sukumara lehya: 2 tsp. with warm milk after breakfast.
- It corrects the menstrual cramps, stimulates the function of uterus.

Ashokarishta: 30 ml after breakfast and dinner.
- Reduces the menstrual cramps, hot flushes, Progesterone effect.

Externally:

Dhanwantara oil Pichu (dipping cotton in oil and applying warm on abdomen relieves menstrual cramps).

HYPERTENSION

- Hypertension is elevated blood pressure: more than 140/90 mm hg.

Symptoms

- Uneasiness or discomfort in the heart region
- Increased sweating
- Anger
- Altered consciousness
- Weight gain.

Ayurveda approach

- One has to maintain proper sleep time and sleep for 7 to 8 hours.
- One has to be calm, avoid angry situations, stress.
- One has to do more meditation (*Dhyana*) and sleeping posture (*Shavasana*), better before breakfast, before work, and before dinner.
- One has also do *Aniloma villoma: Pranayama*.
- One has to drink water mixed with Vetiver roots.
- One has to take grape juice, watermelon, banana, dark chocolates.
- Avoid fatty, oily, fried, salty food.

Ayurveda medicines like

Sarpagandha vati: 2 tablets after dinner

- Relaxes the blood supply to nerves to brain, heart; reduces the blood pressure
- It is not advisable to give more than 2 tablets a day, it may cause giddiness.

Arjunarishta: 30 ml after breakfast and dinner

- Heart tonic, maintains the blood pressure.

Draksharishta: 30 ml after breakfast and dinner

- Protects the heart, increases the oxygenation to the heart hence maintains the blood pressure.

External therapies:

- One should apply *Ksira bala taila, Himasagara taila* as it increases blood supply to brain, relieves tension of blood supply from brain to heart.
- *Shirodhara.*

LOW BACK ACHE

Symptoms

- Pain only in the low back or radiating pain from the low back to either of legs or both.
- Low back maybe to different conditions like: Intervertebral Disc prolapse
- Lumbar spondylitis
- Lumbar canal stenosis
- Lumbago

Ayurveda approach

- To reduce the pain, stiffness.
- To remove the compression of the nerve.

Ayurveda medicines like

Rasnasaptakam Kashaya: 20 ml of decoction with warm water before breakfast and dinner.

- Best medicine to reduce the pain, inflammation in the, low back, spine, waist, hip region.

Gandharvahastadi Kashaya: 20 ml of decoction with warm water before breakfast and dinner.

- It helps to lubricate the back as well as reduce the pain, inflammation in the back.

Trayodashanga guggulu: 2 tablets after breakfast and dinner.

- It has special action on the low back, hip region to reduce the pain, inflammation.

Nirgundi eranadadi taila: 20 ml with hot water bed time once in a week

- It helps in reducing the compression in the low back region

External

- *Sahacharadi taila*
- *Dhanwanatara taila*

Refer Fig 3.2

OBESITY

Symptoms

- Increased body weight more than 6 kgs in one year.
- Body Mass Index: more than 25.
- Deposition of extra weight in the waist, hip, trunk, thigh, face regions.

- On slight exertion feeling breathlessness.
- Fatigue.
- Lethargy whole day.
- Sleep apnea

Ayurveda approach

Diet

- Garcinia indica fruits soaked in water over night and to take it empty morning.
- Fenugreek seeds soaked in water over night and to take it empty morning.
- Cinnamon powder 2 tsp. with honey 2 tsp.
- Lemon juice with hot water.
- Bottle gourd juice.
- Green gram soup.
- Water boiled and reduced to ¾ th quantity.
- Avoid rice items, oily items, baked items, caked food, pastries, confectionaries, ice cream, curd, red meat.
- To reduce fat metabolism, reduce weight by diet and excerise.

Ayurveda medicines like

Varasanadi Kashaya: 20 ml of decoction with warm water before breakfast and dinner.

Varanadi Kashaya: 20 ml of decoction with warm water before breakfast and dinner.

Navaka guggulu: 2 tablets after breakfast and dinner.

Ayaskrti: 30 ml of decoction after breakfast and dinner.

Asanadi Kashaya: 20 ml of decoction with warm water before breakfast and dinner.

The above said medicines helps to scrape, liquify, reduce the body fat and help in fat metabolism.

Refer Fig 3.3

DEPRESSION

Symptoms

- Feeling sad and weak.
- Unable to face small tough situations.
- Inability to concentrate.
- Disturbed sleep, difficulty to fall asleep or interrupted sleep.
- Restlessness during the day.
- Hopelessness or loss of confidence.
- Lack of social interaction, feeling to be alone.

Ayurveda approach

- Activation of mind, strengthening the mind.
- Calming the mind, bringing stability to the mind.
- Social interaction among family, friends.
- One should adore and practice more spirituality in life.
- One should visit churches, temples, mosques regularly.
- Chanting "Om "many times a day (It brings more inner strength, power and stability to the mind).
- Listening to music like melodious songs, classical songs.

- Aroma therapy like lavender oil, jasmine oil in the room.
- One should involve more in reading, painting.

Ayurveda medicines like

Ashwagandharishta: 30 ml of decoction after breakfast and dinner
- Very good nerve tonic to mind, strengthens the mind, stablises the mind and thoughts.

Kalyanaka Ghrita: 5 ml empty stomach
- Strengthens and nourishes the mind, brings clarity to thoughts, promotes intelligence.

Brahmi Ghrita: 5 ml empty stomach
- Strengthens the brain and promotes thinking wisdom

Brahmi vati: 2 tablets after breakfast and dinner

External application

Kachoradi choorna: apply on head
- It acts on brain, releasing tension on nerves, helping depression.

    Ksira bala taila

    Brahmi taila
- Both oils are good for calming, stabilizing the mind, thoughts, intelligence.

Refer Fig 3.4

YOUNG AGE RELATED DISEASES

- WORM INFESTATION 181
- RESPIRATORY TRACT DISEASE 182
- FOOD POISONING 182

YOUNG AGE RELATED DISEASES

WORM INFESTATION

- Children tend to eat more sweets and also play in dirt which leads to entry of microorganisms into the digestive tract.
- This in turn leads to symptoms like stomach pain, lack of appetite, loose stools, itching in anal region.

Ayurveda approach

- Food need to be hygienic
- The child should be kept away from dirt.
- Food with bitter and astringent taste should be given in small quantities eg: Bitter gourd, okra, Spinach, Lettuce, Amaranth should be cooked properly and given.
- Avoid sweet and chocolates.

Ayurveda medicines like

- Dose may change according to age of the child, nothing is specific.
- Krimighna vati: one after breakfast.
- Nimbadi vati: one after breakfast.
- Vidangarishta: 5 ml with warm water after breakfast.

RESPIRATORY TRACT DISEASE

- Respiratory diseases are very common in young age
- Reasons like premature birth, Poor immunity, Poor hygiene, Lack of nutritious food may give rise to these problems
- Symptoms like cough (dry/wet), Running nose, Difficulty in breathing are seen.

Ayurveda approach

- Proper care during pregnancy and post-delivery both of mother and child is to be taken.
- Exposure to dust, cold, poor hygiene, poor food nutrients should be avoided.
- Warm and light food need to be given during the attacks.

Ayurveda medicines like

- Sitopaladi choora with honey: ½ tsp. twice or thrice daily.
- Talisadi choora with honey: ½ tsp. twice or thrice daily.
- Elaadi lehya: ½ tsp. once or twice daily.
- Dashamoolarishta: 5 ml twice or thrice daily.

FOOD POISONING

- Food poisoning caused by eating unhygienic, heavy food, untimely food, lot of milk products and sweets.
- Symptoms like stomach pain, fever, vomiting, and Diarrhea.

Ayurveda approach

- The digestive system of children is very weak to digest heavy food.
- So children should be fed with light, timely, easily digestive food.

Ayurveda medicines like

- Madiphala Rasayana: 5 ml twice or thrice daily.
- Bilwadi gutika: 1 tablet per day.
- Mustakarishta: 5 ml twice or thrice daily.

COMPLETE HEALTH CARE

- SKIN CARE   187
- HAIR CARE   192
- JOINT CARE   198
- DIABETIC CARE   199
- HEART CARE   203
- PREGNANCY CARE   206
- BABY CARE/CHILD CARE   214
- OCCUPATIONAL CARE   217
- WEIGHT LOSS PLAN   220
- POSTURE RELATED PROBLEMS   228
- CLIMATE RELATED BODY PROBLEMS   230

COMPLETE HEALTH CARE

SKIN CARE

- Isn't it everybody's dream to have a beautiful clear skin?
- Skin is the outermost part of our body, and is more exposed to outer atmosphere like sun, wind, dust, cold temperature, hot temperature
- Hence it tends to be more sensitive.
- Skin and blood are directly related.
- When the blood is affected, the skin also loses its quality.

Even the health of skin depends on factors like

1 Food

- The more unhealthy food habits we follow, the more bad would be the skin.
- If we eat spicier, fried, oil the skin tends to be more sensitive and effected by Acne, Eczema, and oily skin.
- If a person eats more alkaline diet like sour, vinegar, baking powder mixed food stuffs, the skin is effected by more dryness, gets cracked, wrinkles appears soon.

2 Sleep

- If sleep habits are untimely then it would reflect on the skin, looking dull, it loses its color or shine.

3 Habits (smoking, alcohol etc.)

- Smoking and drinking habits would affect the skin as it has lot of chemical contents in it, which would make the skin more pigmented.
- Skin gets aged soon; it loses shine, looks tired, worn and torn.

4 Mental status

- When a person is happy it directly reflects on one's skin.
- Ones face becomes brighter, skin appears shiny.
- In the same way if the person is mentally disturbed, then adverse effect is seen on the skin color as it becomes dull or pale, shine fades away.

5 Hormonal imbalance

- When the hormone loses its balance during teenage, there will be Acne or Pimples.
- Whereas during the menopausal stage the skin loses its color, gets hyper pigmented on the skin.

6 Age factor

- During young age as *Kapha dosha* is predominant; children will have allergic rashes with itching.
- Since they are more exposed to dirt, they also get hand, foot, mouth diseases, ring worm etc.
- During middle age, *Pitha dosha* is predominant thus there will be Acne or Pimples, Eczema other skin conditions.
- During old age as *Vata dosha* is predominant the skin becomes dry loses its shine, texture becomes dry, wrinkled, cracked.

Measures to purify skin

Main aims are to

- Purify blood
- As skin and blood are related, the first measure should be taken is to purify blood.

Food best for skin like

- Vegetables like
- Beetroot, carrot, cucumber, tomatoes, bitter gourd, snake gourd, lettuce, spinach, broccoli, coriander leaves, dark leafy vegetables, mint leaves, fennel leaves etc.
- Fruits especially the ones having Vitamin C like strawberries, raspberries, lemon, orange, grape, kiwi, Indian goose berry, pomegranate, papaya, Apricot, avocados etc.
- Nuts like almond, hazel nut, pistachios in limited quantity.
- Fish like sardine, king fish, silver fish, salmon, anchovies, herring, seer fish.

Avoid food and drinks

- Food like salty, sour, spicy should be avoided.
- Food stuffs which are fried, baked, preserved like burgers, pizzas, chips, bacon are also bad for skin.
- Vegetables like brinjal, asparagus, and ladies finger.
- Fruits like chikku, pineapple, are not good for skin.
- Meat like red meats and fishes like mackerel, shrimps, oysters, and cuttle fish should be avoided.
- Beverages like alcohol, beer, coke or carbonated drinks, coffee are the worst for skin.

- Avoid exposure to extreme environment.
- Exposure to the sun after 12 pm–3 pm is very harmful for the skin as the sun rays will be very stronger. Hence it is better to avoid this time.
- Exposure to dust, cold wind, damp areas etc are to be avoided.
- Perform *Yoga* or *Pranayama* which increases circulation over head and face.
- *Yoga* like sun salutation, *Bhujangasana* (cobra pose), *Balasana* (child pose), *Shashankasana* (rabbit pose), *Halasana* (plough pose).
- Pranayama like *Kapalabathi, Bastrika, Seetali, Sitkari, Anuloma viloma.*
- Exercises like walking, jogging, aerobics are good for the skin.

Ayurveda medicine

Manjistadi kashaya: 20 ml before breakfast and dinner with warm water

Patola katu rohinyadi kashaya: 20 ml before breakfast and dinner with warm water

Shonitamrutha Kashaya: 20 ml before breakfast and dinner with warm water

Araghwadhadi kashaya: 20 ml before breakfast and dinner with warm water

Khadirarishta: 30 ml after breakfast and dinner.

Tiktaka Ghrita: 2 tsp. after dinner

Maha tiktaka Ghrita: 2 tspn. after dinner

Gandhaka rasayana: 2 tablets after breakfast and dinner.

All these medicines purify the blood, help in reducing itching and other skin problems.

Facial paste like

- *Nalpmaradi lepam*
- *Manjishtadi lepam*

Few Ayurveda oils best for skin problems like

- *Nalpamaradi oil*
- *Marichadi oil*
- *Eladi oil*
- *Dinesha vilvadi oil*

Face packs or mask to beautify your skin

- Paste of Turmeric with coconut milk or raw milk should be applied over the face and body and kept for 30 min for a better skin.
- Cucumber juice applied on face and kept for 15 min, helps to reduce sun tan, pigmentations, and dark spots.
- Neem paste should be applied over the face .It reduces acne, itching and infection.
- Orange peel powder with chick pea's flour should be made into paste using rose water and applied over the skin.
- It should be kept for drying and washed with warm water .It helps to reduce the excess oiliness from the skin and acne.
- Orange peel powder with cream of milk should be applied over the face and left for 20 min It helps the skin to have a radiant color and glow.
- Yogurt applied plainly or with turmeric helps to get rid of dry skin and acts as natural bleach.

- Tomato paste applied on the skin helps lighten the facial hairs and provides good skin glow.
- Honey applied over the face is best bleach, improves skin glow.

Refer Fig 3.5

HAIR CARE

Good hairs, good hairstyle and texture of hairs is the prime attraction of one's looks.

It is everybody's wish to have thick and good hairs.

Types of hair

- Dry hair
- Oily hair
- Moderate hairs

Dry hairs

- Person with *Vata dosha* will mainly have curly, rough, little quantity, frizzy hairs.
- Scalp will be affected by dandruff or itching.

Causes of increased scalp dryness

- Food like bread, biscuits, baked items, increased nuts intake.
- Activities like travelling, irregular and untimely sleep patterns.
- Emotional disturbances like anxiety, increased stress, washing hairs with chemical based
- Shampoos, using hot water for hair wash.

Measures to moisten and strengthen hair

Food

- Food with taste like sweet and sour is to be taken.
- Green leafy vegetables like spinach, amaranth, lettuce.
- Fruits like banana, pomegranate, and papaya.
- Intake of milk, milk products, ghee.
- Egg and meat, in moderate quantities.
- Fishes like sardine, king fish, salmon, tuna are good for having healthy hairs.
- Avoid intake salty, spicy like chilies, alkaline like vinegar, baking soda
- Daily application of oil on scalp, washing hairs with Luke warm water.

Few tips for dry and rough hair

Heat the coconut oil slightly, add curry leaves to it and apply warm on scalp with good massage.

- Would smoothen, reduce dandruff, thicken, and strengthen the hair roots and delays graying of hairs.

Heat coconut oil with cumin seeds and apply warm on scalp

- Would smoothen the hair, impart a good texture and color to the hair and maintain the scalp temperature.

Paste of curds and egg yolk should be applied on scalp and left for one hour and then washed.

- It would smoothen hair texture, reduce dandruff and hair fall problems.

Leaves and flower of Hibiscus is made into paste and applied on scalp about half an hour before bath.

- It is a best moisturizer for hair as it smoothens the hair, reduces the hair fall and increases hair growth.

Leaves of hibiscus, flower, cumin, and fenugreek are heated in coconut oil, later filtered.

- This oil is best for hair growth as it removes the roughness of hair, reduces itching and reduces hair fall.

Aloe Vera pulp is applied on scalp with egg yolk and applied on scalp.

It should be kept for half an hour.

- It is best hair moisturizer, reduces dandruff problems, itchy scalp and reduces hair fall.

Oily hair

- The person with increased *Pitha* and *Kapha dosha* will have oily and wet hairs.
- The scalp will be affected by wet dandruff, small eruptions and itchy scalp.

Causes of oily hair

- Increased food intake of oily, fried, fat rich food increases the oiliness of the scalp and hair.
- Increased sweat also makes the hair wet all the time and hair will be having foul smell.
- Person with increased anger, emotional disturbances will be commonly affected by this.

Measures to reduce the stickiness and oiliness of hairs

- Food with light quality like wheat, oats, barley, puffed corns, nuts should be taken.
- Food that cools down the increased heat like juices of grapes, lemon, berries, coconut water, and water melon should be consumed.
- Avoid exposure to excess heat and avoid over stress of the body and mind.
- Avoid application of oil on the scalp.
- Wash hairs almost daily with water having room temperature (not cold).

Few tips to reduce stickiness or wet hair

Apply the paste of henna on hair. Leave it for 1 hour and rinse it off.

- It helps to reduce the sticky dandruff, reduce the heat of scalp and helps in strengthening the hair roots.

Apply the paste of Indian goose berry. Leave it for 1 hour and rinse it off.

- It helps to reduce the oiliness and stickiness of hairs, helps in increased hair growth, gives good texture to the hair.

Chick pea's powder made into paste with water and applied on the scalp and kept for 1 hour and rinsed off.

- It helps in giving a best texture to the hair and removes the excess oil in hair.

Basil leaves along with paste of henna should be applied on the scalp.

- It helps in scrapping off the sticky dandruff and helps to get rid of the itchy scalp. It also reduces hair fall and enhances the hair growth.

General tips to maintain hair conditions

Do's

- Wash hair once in 2 days, wash with Luke warm water.
- Always use herbal based shampoo products.
- Apply oil on the scalp daily and let it remain (in dry hair), for oily hairs one may apply oil once in a week and wash it after 10–15 min.
- Hairs should be dried completely after bath.
- Maintain hygiene of the comb, bathing towel, pillow covers.
- People, who travel more, should cover ones hairs with a cotton cloth.
- This prevents exposure towards extreme conditions like wind, sunlight which are causative factors of hair fall.

Don'ts

- Don't use chemical based shampoo daily.
- Don't comb wet hair or don't tie wet hairs.
- Don't wash hairs late night or late evening.
- Don't follow unhealthy sleep habits and food habits.
- Don't expose to excess cold, sunlight, dust and extreme conditions.

Medicines for healthy hair

Internal medicine

Chyavanaprasha: 2 tsp. after breakfast with milk

- It is a wonderful medicine for hair care, for skin and general immunity as it contains herbs having rejuvinative and antioxidant property.

Brahma rasayana: 2 tsp. after breakfast with milk

- It is the best neuro oxidative medicine which helps in preventing premature graying as well as hair fall.

Narasimha rasayana: 2 tsp. after breakfast

- It is the best medicine for initiating hair growth and strengthening the hair roots.
- It is better to be avoided in persons with *Pitha dosha* predominance and *Pitha dosha* related disorders. As it increases male characteristics, it should be taken in caution by women.

Bhringarajaasava: 30 ml after breakfast and dinner

- It is very good nutritional supplement for hair growth, a very good liver tonic and good rejuvinative medicine.

External application

Nila bhringadi oil

- It is very good to strengthen the hair rootlets, increases hair growth, removes dandruff, best in premature graying of hairs.

Brahmi oil

- It is very good for hair growth, cools the scalp, gives good sleep.

Dhurdhurapatradi oil

- It is best in case of dandruff, itchy scalp or Foliiculitis.

Asana manjishtadi oil

- In people with Cold, Rhinitis, Migraine, this oil gives best result.

Refer Fig 3.6

JOINT CARE

Joint are the basic support of the body. The joints are made up of various structures like bones, muscles, tendons, ligaments.

Joints are responsible for stability, yet they are sensitive to any kind of injury, inflammation, degeneration as well as calcification.

The most commonly affected joint diseases are Rheumatoid arthrittis

- Osteo arthrittis
- Gouty arthrittis
- Fracture of joints

Main aim

The main aim is to prevent the diseases; hence one has to maintain healthy food and lifestyle in order to maintain healthy joints.

Food and medications which can strengthen the joints.

Foods: Food having bitter and sweet taste is good for the joints.

- Food having qualities like hot, smoothness.
- Vegetables like spinach, amaranth, long green beans, broccoli, lettuce, basil leaves, mint leaves, carrot, beet root, ash gourd, melons.
- Wheat, brown rice, ragi, muesli.
- Fruits like pomegranate, banana, grapes, fig, plums, berries, pears.
- Cow's milk, soy milk, almond milk.
- Meat like mutton, lamb, wild chicken.
- Sea food sardine, tuna, king fish, salmon, silver fish.
- Nuts like cashew, almond, hassle nuts, peanut in moderate quantity. Over eating of nuts causes dryness in the body and joints.
- Activities like walking, swimming, Yoga is advisable.

DIABETIC CARE

- Diabetes reminds of sweets.
- People have a misconception that just by avoiding sweets the sugar level would come into control which is not the truth.
- Diabetes is a lifestyle disorder along with a little possibility of genetics.
- According to Ayurveda, main reasons for diabetes is always sitting or sedentary lifestyle, always lying down or sleeping.
- Following irregular timings of food, eating more fat rich food like curds, meat, fried food are the other reasons.

Management

- Lifestyle modification is mainly required which would give best results.
- One should be engaged with activities, and be more active.
- Avoid sitting postures for long time; one should not sleep in the daytime.

Yogasana

Morning *Yogasana a*re best like *Shashankasna* (rabbit pose), *Bhujanghasana* (cobra posture), *Halasana* (plough pose), *Naukasana (*boat posture).

- Person who has their profession with more of sitting posture it is unavoidable to insist them not to do.
- They instead can engage rest of their time with exercises and evening walks.
- Evening walk is best for Diabetic patients. One should walk for about 45–60 min in the evening.

Food

- Eat small frequent meals as Diabetic patients will have more hunger and chances of sudden drop down in sugar levels are high.
- Eat more quantity of barley, moderate quantity of wheat products, oats.
- Cut off carbohydrate rich food like rice.
- One should include more of bitter and astringent taste food in diet like bitter gourd, okra.
- One should eat very less quantity of fruits.
- Indian gooseberry, guava, moderately ripened papaya can be taken.
- Avoid milk products, meat, and frozen, tinned, preserved food.
- Avoid fat rich food like pastries, junk, fried, sweets.
- Turmeric is a very good spice to maintain blood sugar level as well a very good anti-oxidant.
- Turmeric with Indian gooseberry is the best remedy for controlling the blood sugar level as well as preventing urinary infection. It provides instant energy.
- Cinnamon powder is helpful to lower high blood sugar level.
- Fenugreek seeds, aloe Vera, ivory gourd, snake gourd, jamun seeds.
- Bottle gourd, barley.

Medicines in Diabetes

Nishamalaki powder: 2 teaspoon with glass of warm water after lunch

- Maintains blood glucose levels, provides anti-oxidants hence relieving tiredness.

Chandraprabha vati: 2 tablets after breakfast and lunch

- Maintains the flow of urine, normalizes the blood glucose levels, and provides rejuvenation to the cells.

Triphala choorna

- It is very good antioxidant, corrects the blood glucose levels.
- It prevents Diabetes complications like Diabetes retinopathy

Nishakathakadi Kashaya

Kathakakhadiradi Kashaya

- Dose: 20 ml with warm water before breakfast and before dinner.
- Both *Kashaya* activates insulin secretion, purifies urine as well as blood.
- It also reduces the turbidity of urine.

Guduchi satva: 2 tsp. with one glass of water after breakfast and dinner.

- This medicine helps to purify the liver as well as pancreas.
- It helps to build immunity as well as prevents early degeneration of the body.
- Herbs like *Kalamegha, Meshashringi, Lajjalu, Punarnava* etc are best single herbs for alleviating the blood sugar levels.

Diabetic schedule

Time	Activities
6 am	Wake up
	Spend half an hour to freshen up
6:30 am–7:15 am	Warm up exercises
	Yogasana
	Vajrasana (diamond pose), *(Paschimothasana)*,
	Balasana (Child pose),
	sun salutation 4/5 rounds
	breathing exercise (Pranayam)
	Anuloma viloma
	Sheetali
7:20 am–7:40 am	*Sitkari*
	walking
8:30 am	Breakfast
12:30 pm	Lunch
4:30 pm	Snacks
5:30 pm–6:00 pm	Walking
7:30 pm	Dinner
10:00 pm/10:30 pm	Go to bed

Diabetic diet

Break fast	Lunch	Snacks	Dinner
1. Oats cooked with water Green tea	Broken wheat (should be roasted) cooked Butter milk (diluted) Radish salad	Puffed corn Green tea	Chapathi (dry) with steamed vegetables
2. Semolina cooked with water Black plum juice	Green gram kichadi Capsicum salad	Stuffed chapathi	Mixed vegetable soup.

Diabetic diet			
Break fast	**Lunch**	**Snacks**	**Dinner**
3. Barley cooked with water Lemon juice with salt	Wheat pan cake Tomato onion salad	Special Sandwich Cucumber juice	Mushroom soup Wheat pancake
4. Semolina vegetable mix Banana stem juice	Mint leaves soup Diabetic rice	Guava 2 in no	Tomato soup
5. Corn flakes with diluted milk Cocum juice	Cucumber onion salad	Green gram salad Black plum	Mint leaf soup

HEART CARE

- Heart is the major organ responsible for life. The heart supplies blood to all other parts of the body.
- Heart is the organ which should be mainly taken care.
- When we express any emotion we touch our heart, it means that emotions and heart are related.
- When a person is emotionally disturbed he feels uncomfortable in the heart region i.e.
- The heart rate varies and it is felt by the person.
- Stress physically or mentally affects the heart.
- Few people may be hyperactive who want to do and get things done soon.
- Few people are such who get anger and aggressive very soon.
- Few people may have a very negative thinking where they even turn cool situation into worst situation.

- All these people are easily prone to heart diseases.
- Other side High blood pressure, hyper cholesterol, heart attack, plaque formation in the heart are the commonly affected heart conditions.

Main aim is to maintain healthy condition of heart

- One should maintain a calm mind as well as positive attitude.
- One should also avoid anger, over stress and emotions, in order to maintain healthy heart.
- Food choice should be a special concern for heart patients.

Do's

- Wheat, oats, corn.
- Vegetables and spices like beetroot, carrot, ash gourd, melons, capsicum, lady's finger, lettuce, broccoli, onion, garlic, ginger, and cinnamon.
- Fruits like pomegranate, grapes, mango, avocadoes, watermelon, all berries, orange, lemon, Indian gooseberry, cocum, tamarind.
- Meat of wild chicken, turkey, duck. Avoid red meat like mutton, beef, pork.
- Meat in the form of barbeque is best.
- Sea food sardine, tuna, king fish, salmon, silver fish.
- Person should build up a positive and cool approach towards all situations.

Don'ts

- Yoga like *Shashankasana* (rabbit pose), *Makarasana* (crocodile pose), *Vajrasana* (diamond pose), *Pavana muktasana* (air releasing pose).
- *Pranayama* like *Nadi shuddi, Sheetali, Sitkari* should be practiced would help In strengthening the heart.

- Meditation should be practiced at least twice a day to balance stress and control emotions.
- There is a telling that if mind is happy heart too will be happy.
- So person should engage himself with his favorite hobbies like gardening, travelling, music, etc which makes mind more calm and stable.
- Interacting with family members as well as friends about his day to day activities and experiences would bring lot of changes in thinking.
- It also would remove frustration, sense of hopelessness and brings about positivity.
- Hence it will help in having healthy, strong heart.

Ayurveda medicine

Arjunarishta: 30 ml after breakfast and dinner.

- It is a cardio tonic, thus it improves blood circulation to the heart.

Drakshadi Kashaya: 20 ml with warm water before breakfast and before dinner.

- It is sour and sweet; hence it enhances the heart function and protects the heart.

Lashunadi Kashaya: 20 ml with warm water before breakfast and before dinner.

- It is very beneficial in person having heart problem (heart block) associated with elevated cholesterol levels.

Guugulutikataka Kashaya: 20 ml with warm water before breakfast and before dinner.

- It scrapes as well as prevents the plaque formation in the heart vessels.
- It also helps it cutting down the excess body fat.

Sarpagandha vati: 2 tablets after breakfast and lunch.

- It helps in reducing the blood pressure by strengthening the nerves and relaxing the nerve tension.

Rasonadi vati: 2 tablets after breakfast and lunch.

- It is very effective in plaque formation, reduces the cholesterol level and corrects the digestive problems.

Dadimadi lehya: 2 tsp. after breakfast.

- It is sour and sweet in taste; hence it enhances the heart function, protects and strengthens the heart.

PREGNANCY CARE

- Pregnancy care includes care of both the pregnant lady and the fetus.
- According to Ayurveda, the pregnancy care starts before the conception.
- If the conceived fetus must be healthy, then both parents need to follow healthy regimen.
- Pregnancy care can be divided into two,

1 Pre conception

- The physical as well as mental health of man and woman is essential for a healthy baby.
- Both partners need to undergo a complete health checkup especially reproductive health.
- Males need to undergo Semen analysis.

- Females need to undergo USG abdomen and a Thyroid profile.
- Sex should not be a mechanical way to have a child.
- It should be done with happiness with utmost love and concern towards each other.
- One should follow healthy sexual habits.
- In the present stressful environment both partners need to find balance between professional and sexual life.
- Food habits are also equally important for a healthy conception.
- One should eat more homely food; avoid junk, spicy, fried food.
- One should include more vegetarian diet in pre conceptional period.
- Food should include more of vegetables, fruits, juices, which help in rejuvenation.
- E.g.: Milk, ghee, egg, pomegranate, grapes, jackfruit, dates, banana, saffron, cumin seeds, ladies finger, Indian gooseberry, muesli.
- Meat like beef, pork, wild chicken, fish should be taken but in less quantity.
- The partners should undergo Purification or Detoxification therapy before conception.
- For females, Vomiting therapy is advised.
- For males Purgation therapy is advised with suitable medications.
- Milk and ghee (plain form) should be included as a daily drink as it builds up the immunity.
- It is rejuvinative, vitalizer and sexual enhancer.

Few Ayurvedic medicines for females:
- Ghee preparations

Dadimadi Ghrita

- This is given in order to nourish the blood tissue, improves digestion, especially best treatment in infertility, and prevents abortions and miscarriages.

Sukumara Ghrita

- It strengthens the female reproductive organs, enhances sexual capacity of both males and females.

For males,

Ashwagandhadi lehya

- It increases the sperm count and motility as well as Testosterone hormone.

Amrtha prasha Ghrita

- It corrects Infertility, or loss of libido.

And many other formulations can be used to maintain health or reproductive system and result in healthy conception.

2 Conception

- When the partners unite the sperm and ovum meets together and conception occurs
- Signs of conception according to Ayurveda,
- Increased salivation, heaviness all over the body especially in breasts, tiredness, and goose bumps.
- There will be absence of menstruation, pain in the nipples and darkening of it.
- Nausea and vomiting, cramping, increased urination will also be present.
- Cravings for sour food.
- Food like light, digestive food like milk porridge, rice water, rice with ghee, cumin seed water, pomegranate, grapes.

3 Post conception (Antenatal care)

- Pregnant women who desire to give birth to a healthy child must follow healthy food habits and certain regimen or activities.

Surroundings and room:

- Pleasant atmosphere.
- Presence of partner and behavior of him should be pleasing.
- Pregnant lady should engage herself with her favorite hobby.
- She also should engage in spiritual activities.
- She should wear comfortable clothing which is not too tight.
- She should have an oil massage herself with mild pressure and take bath daily.
- She should use chairs, bed or furniture which is soft and comfortable and bed with head rest slightly elevated.
- Food should be hygienic and healthy.
- Food like tasty, liquid, sweet, protein rich, appetizers need to be eaten.
- One should take milk diet as it nourishes the fetus and brings stability to the fetus. Hence it avoids miscarriage.
- Food like ghee, rice, green gram, wheat, honey, banana, Indian goose berry, yogurt, grapes or raisins are to be taken as it stabilizes the increased *Vata dosha* and *Pitha dosha*.
- If *Vata dosha* and *Pitha dosha* is imbalanced, it is harmful for the pregnancy.
- It leads to increased chances of miscarriage and mal nourishment of the fetus.
- Month wise diet is advised in Ayurveda so that the fetus develops best and it builds good immunity and strength.

First month of pregnancy

Diet for first month of pregnancy	Therapy
The conceived matter should remain and nourish so nourishing food should be taken.	Oil massage With *Dhanwantara* oil
Milk should be consumed in more quantity as per the digestive capacity of a person. Increased quantity may cause indigestion.	Pouring of *Dashamoola* decoction all over the body
	Pouring of oil all over the body.
	Oil like *Ksheerabala* oil, *Balaashwagandha* oil.
First twelve days of conception, ghee is to be consumed.	Internal medications which eliminates excess *Vata dosha*, *Jeerakadi Kashaya*, *Dashamoola Kashaya* with milk,
Water boiled with gold/silver is drunk after milk consumption.	For nausea and vomiting along with tiredness and loss of appetite *Madhiphala rasayana* is one of the best.
It helps the milk to reach the target and act at its best.	
Fruits like banana, watermelon, pomegranate, grapes, and figs.	
Vegetables like beetroot, carrot, broccoli, lettuce.	

Second month of pregnancy

Diet for second month of pregnancy	Therapy
Milk processed with sweet things like liqorice.	Same as first month
Liquid food like rice water	In addition
The food with cool potency like Vetivera root water.	*Shatavari ksheera Kashaya*: it acts as rejuvinator, nourishes the uterus and body.
Appetizers like cumin seed in food and water.	*Dhanwanatara* pills with hot water.
	It removes constipation or gas troubles.
Avoid spicy, bitter, astringent variety of food.	*Matulunga rasayana* for vomiting and morning sickness.
Fruits like banana, grapes, lemon.	
Vegetables like beans, spinach, amaranth, cucumber.	

Third month of pregnancy

Diet	Therapy
Milk rich diet.	Same therapy as first and second month
Diet with cool property.	
Milk with honey and ghee (take honey and ghee in different proportions)	
Rice cooked with milk and sweetening agents (jaggery or sugar candy).	
One should take fruits like banana, orange, pomegranate, watermelon.	
Vegetables like carrot, cucumber, melons, ash gourd, and pumpkin.	

Fourth month of pregnancy

Diet	Therapy
Butter is to be eaten in specific quantity as it nourishes the fetus and mother and cools body.	Oil massage with *Dhanwantara* oil.
Curd rice should be eaten	There may be constipation so one should take *Sukumara ghritha*, *Dhanwantara* pills.
Food or rice mixed with milk. Butter, meat soup.	Hemoglobin may decrease so iron content pills like *Dhatri loha* is effective.
Food liked by the pregnant women or desired food	*Punarnava mandoora* can also be taken.

Fifth month of pregnancy

Diet	Therapy
Ghee extracted from	
Rice cooked with milk	
Meat soup	

Sixth month of pregnancy

Diet	Therapy
Ghee extracted from milk should be processed with sweet substances, like sugar candy, and jaggery.	
Sweet substances are to be included in the diet like deserts, juices and fruits rich diet.	
Curd mixed with honey, jaggery or sugar candy can be taken.	

Seventh month of pregnancy

Diet	Therapy
Same as that of sixth month	

Eight month of pregnancy

Diet	Therapy
Rice cooked with milk is to be consumed.	Enema is administered with oil, honey, ghee, milk and other herbs.
Ghee and milk should be taken in sufficient quantity.	It helps to remove Constipation, obstructed gas in the intestine.
Meat soup should be taken.	

Ninth month of pregnancy

Diet	Therapy
Meat soup cooked with rice and ghee should be consumed.	Vaginal tamponing with oil is done in order to lubricate the uterus, vaginal canal and cervix.
Rice porridge with ghee should be taken.	Enema should be given with oil, and other herbs.
	Women with dry skin should apply oil to body and take bath with herbs having old potency like sandal wood, Vetivera roots etc.

Significance of following the diet and therapy during each month of pregnancy is,

- By above said measures the reproductive canal like vaginal canal, cervix, abdomen, hip region, becomes stronger and softer.
- Thus the air moves in downward direction making easy urine, stool output. Hence it results in easy delivery without complications.
- By following all these properly women gains complexion, strength, good health, and long life.
- There will be adequate breast, nipple development and milk production will be normal.

Things to be avoided by pregnant women

- Food with pungent taste, hot properties, and increased meat intake should be avoided.
- One should not eat dried up, pale, stale food.
- One should strictly avoid alcohol and smoking.
- One should avoid sexual intercourse, heavy exercise, and major *Panchakarma* procedure.
- One should avoid controlling urge of urination and stools.
- Places which are unhygienic or dirty places, foul smelling are to be avoided.
- Travelling, violent activities, running etc. should be avoided.
- High pitch talks, anger, crying, sadness, being alone are to be avoided.
- All these activities may hamper the stability of fetus, thus leading to miscarriage or abortion.
- It may cause deformity in the fetus or may cause complications during or after delivery both to the mother and child.

BABY CARE/CHILD CARE

"Strength of the building lies in its foundation"

- A healthy baby will grow into a strong adult.
- Journey of a baby starts right from the mother's womb.
- Pregnancy care is equally important and thus contributes a major role in deciding the health of a baby.
- For a healthy journey of life, a strong body with a strong immune system is a necessity.
- According to Ayurveda, different rituals/measures are performed during the different stages of baby's life.

Day of birth

- It starts right from the umbilical cord separation.
- Here the baby's nutritional supplement from mother's cord is separated, so the baby becomes dependent on other sources for nutrition.
- Sudden change in the environment from womb to external atmosphere creates changes in the baby.
- Baby has to undergo many changes.
- If proper measures are not taken during this time, the baby may become weak.

Gold immunity booster drops

- The small blunt stick about 1–2 inches made up of gold, is dipped in a mixture of ghee and honey with several herbs in less quantity.
- Ghee and honey taken in unequal quantity should be dropped on the tongue of the baby.
- 2 drop in just born baby to 1 year.

- 4 drops from 1 year and above up to 14 years.
- It is better to give for continuous 24 months for maximum benefits.
- It acts like a vaccine or immunity booster which enhances the growth of the baby, nourishes the baby.
- It makes the baby intelligent, healthy skin, color and complexion to the baby.
- It also enhances the power of sense organs, gives good grasping power to the baby.

Breast milk and feeding

- The breast milk of the mother should be fat rich, liquid namely colostrum.
- Breast feeding should be done very carefully.
- First the quantity and quality of breast milk should be observed,
- Few females have adequate and thick breast milk which would be sufficient to feed the baby every 2–3 hours.
- Few of them have less and thin breast milk, by which baby will have insufficient nutrition and which cannot fulfill the baby's hunger.
- For adequate and nutrition rich breast milk, mother should consume few food and medicines.
- Milk and milk products like curds, cheese in moderate quantity.

Few Ayurveda medicines like

- *Shatavari ghritha, Shatavari choorna with milk*
- Mother must avoid food like fried oil, baked, spicy, salty which hampers the quality and quantity of breast milk.
- If there is hardening of breast then slight fomentation on breast can be done.

- Before and after each feed, the mother should wet the nipple and surrounding with warm water and clean it dry with cloth to avoid infection and to maintain hygiene.
- After each feed, mother should gently pat on the baby's back till the baby burps.
- This is very important because if the air remains within the baby's digestive tract, it would hamper digestion and hunger of the baby.

Baby oil massage

- Gentle oil massage should be done to the baby.
- Techniques of oil massage for babies are different as they have very delicate skin, bones, joints.
- Massage should be done by experienced person before the bath.
- After oil massage, baby should be exposed to sunlight with light cotton cloth covered as it is best source for Vitamin D.
- This would enhance bone growth.
- Oil like *Balagraha* oil.

Bathing babies

- Babies should be carefully bathed with warm water (which is pre boiled).
- Care should be taken that water doesn't enter nose, ears, and mouth.
- Water should be boiled with medicinal herbs like *Nalpmara*, *Neem*.

After bath

- The baby is wrapped medium tight with a soft cotton cloth.
- Baby is made to sleep in cradle with soft and clean cotton bed and coverings.

- The cradle and room where baby is placed should be fumigated with herbs like
- *Guggulu, Jatamamsi, Neem, Karpoora, Chandana, Agaru* etc.
- It acts as disinfectant, insect repellent, maintains healthy skin of the baby.
- For premature baby, bathing is not advised as it may affect the body temperature of the baby.
- So a cloth is dipped in warm water and wiped over the baby's body and patted dry.

OCCUPATIONAL CARE

- **High targets!!! Expectations reaching heights!! Competition among colleagues!!**

Aim for short term benefits!!

- What would all these end up with? Stress!! Stress!! Stress!!
- The present stressful occupational conditions lead to physical as well as mental disturbances.
- Jobs related to different fields leads to different health issues.
- Example like in Engineers: back pain, neck pain, Computer stress syndrome, Obesity, Diabetes.

Teachers, Chef, House wife: Varicosity.

Drivers, Pilot: Constipation, Piles.

Businessman, IT Professionals, Marketing officials: Back pain.

Chemical industry: Respiratory problems, Skin problems.

General Approach for good occupational health:

Change your lifestyle!

Make a daily schedule which is easy to do and fix to it.

Daily schedule	
To do	Time
Sleep	6–8 hours
Workout (yoga/walk/jog/cycling)	30–60 min
Meditation	10–20 min

Please note

- Make sure that a person takes short break in between the long working hours, which reduces almost half of stress.
- Short breaks like closing eyes and meditating (2–5 min), speaking to colleagues about things other than work.
- Do not mix up professional and family life!!!
- This is the main cause to add up stress or health problems.
- Home is the place where you can be yourself.
- After reaching home from work, meditate, be calm and relax.
- Forget work stress and later have good talk with spouse, parents and children about your day.
- Speak out or share your daily experience (good or bad), stop showing your frustration on spouse or children. This change would surely keep you pleasant and healthy.
- Take short a vacation once in 2 months (5–7 days), which would give you space to build up your family relationship and would keep you away from work stress.

Ayurveda approach

According to profession the approach slightly differs.

1 People with sedentary jobs like IT Professionals, corporates should mainly concentrate on before and after work activities

- One should have proper sleep, practice meditation and *Yoga Nidra* before work.
- Workouts like walking/jogging/cycling and yoga is advisable.
- It helps to strengthen the stiffened or lazy muscles after long time sitting and computer work.
- It also burns out the excess fat deposited in the belly, hips and buttock.
- *Yoga* like *Tadasana* (palm tree pose or mountain pose), *Ushtrasana* (camel pose), *Setubandhasana* (bridge posture), *Vajrasana* (diamond pose) with mudra.
- It helps to have a flexible spine and reduce pain in the neck and hip.

Ayurveda medicines to prevent diseases caused by sedentary life are

1. *Chyavanprasha*: it increases vitality; it strengthens the stiffened muscles due to wrong postures or long time sitting.
2. *Triphala choorna*: It helps in reducing Obesity, very good anti-oxidant, good for eyes and skin
3. *Nisha amalaki choorna:* very good anti-oxidant.
4. *Ashwagandhadi* capsules: it helps in getting a good sleep, is a nerve tonic, relives stress from the body, and promotes muscle bulk.
5. *Maha Triphaladi Ghrita*: good for eyes and skin.

2 People like teachers, chefs who stand for long should be suggested a very mild workout and a fixed schedule

- The above mentioned people stand for long time; hence pressure is increased over the ankle, knees and foot.
- They should fix the sleeping hours not more than 6–7 hours.

- Mild workout and certain yoga postures are advised to strengthen the leg and foot muscles, increase the blood circulation.
- *Yoga* like *Uttanapadasana* (leg raising posture), *Shirshasana* (head pose), *Halasana* (plough pose) should be practiced.

Ayurveda medicine to prevent Varicosity and other leg related problems are

1. *Sahacharadi kashayam*: it is best for problems related to lower limbs, as it increases the blood circulation, strengthens the muscles, and nerves.
2. *Rasna erandadi kashayam*: it relives the pain, stiffness in muscles and joint related problems, relives constipation and enhances blood circulation.
3. *Pinda taila:* it is best in varicosity or gout related problems, increases the circulation in legs and strengthens the muscles.

Refer Fig 3.7

WEIGHT LOSS PLAN

- To fit into a trendy dress is everybody's dream.
- For this, having a fit and optimum weight is very essential.
- But either due to hereditary factors or bad food habits and lifestyle, a person becomes like a pot.
- Gaining weight is comparatively easy, while losing weight is hard.
- Losing weight is not a sudden process; patience is a key factor.
- Gradual weight loss would be safer, better and easier in terms of health.
- The main aim of doing this is to maintain weight evenly.
- Lifestyle modification, daily exercise, sleep, waking patterns apart from diet is most important.

Sleep	By 10:30 pm
Wake up	By 6:00 am
Work out	Morning hours: 30–45 min (6:30–7/7:15 am)
	Evening hours: 30–45 min (5:30–6/6:15 pm)
	Both in empty stomach
Water intake (per day)	2–3 litres/day
	0.5–1 litres/night
Food intake	Breakfast by 8:30–9 am
	Lunch by 12:30–1:00 am
	Dinner by 7:30–8:00 pm

Days	Food	
Day 1	Breakfast	apple 2 in no.
		Pomegranate 1 in no.
		Honey water
	Lunch	water melon 5–6 slices
		Avocadoes 1 in no.
		Cucumber with mint juice
	Dinner	papaya 5–6 slices
		Pears 1 in no.
Day 2	Breakfast	steamed carrot+ steamed long beans+ lettuce (all together about 250–300 gms)
	Lunch	diced cucumber + beetroot + broccoli
	Dinner	spinach soup
		Capsicum+onion+carrot salad (150–200 gms)
Day 3	Breakfast	papaya, pomegranate, apple fruit salad
		Beetroot juice (with honey)
	Lunch	soup of carrot
		Cucumber, beetroot, sprouts, lettuce salad
		Lemon juice with cardamom powder
	Dinner	steamed vegetables (carrot, long beans) 250–300 gms
		Papaya slices 6–7 in no.

Days	Food	
Day 4	Breakfast	herbal tea
		Oats 1 cup (with boiled vegetables)
	Lunch	beetroot or mixed vegetables soup
		Cinnamon drink
	Dinner	soup of spinach
		Salads of steamed carrot, cabbage, broccoli
Day 5	Banana diet	
	Breakfast	steamed banana 200–250 gms
		2 glass of milk
	Lunch	banana salad
		Garlic milk
	Dinner	carrot soup
		steamed banana 200 gms
Day 6	Breakfast	tomato with onion salad 200–250 gms
		Cucumber juice with honey
	Lunch	tomato soup
		Chapatti (2 in no.): with steamed vegetables
	Dinner	tomato soup
		Steamed vegetables
Day 7	Breakfast	oats with vegetables
		Lemon juice with honey
	Lunch	chapatti (2 in no.) with soya curry
		Salad of carrot, cucumber, capsicum
	Dinner	mixed vegetable soup
		Steamed vegetable salad
Day 8	Breakfast	chapatti (2 in no.) with steamed vegetable
	Lunch	brown rice (200–250 gms)
		Chicken (1 breast piece) steamed without oil
		Or cottage cheese (100 gm)
	Dinner	chapatti (2 in no.) with steamed vegetables
		Papaya 5–6 slices

Mode of action of 8 days weight loss program

Day 1: The diet starts with fruits which is more of hydrating having sweet and sour tastes. This prepares the digestive system for weight loss by providing adequate glucose reserve.

- Thus it avoids dehydration.

Day 2: The body is now prepared for losing weight. So the sweet supplements in terms of fruits are reduced. The diet is switched to fibrous green mineral rich vegetables.

Day 3: Fruits and vegetables are to be eaten to maintain glucose in the body as well as fiber intake.

- Here there is zero salt and sugar intake by which excessive fluid is lost.
- There by the body easily loses its weight.

Day 4: On day 1, 2, 3 the food pattern is fruits and vegetables. Tongue feels monotonous and by this body feels tired. So salads of vegetables and juices are taken.

Day 5: The diet till day 4 has no calcium and protein supplements. This day concentrates on calcium supplement to body.

Day 6: Body now requires qualities of food which can hasten the weight loss process. Tomato being sour and alkaline helps for the same.

Day 7: Diet here is mixture of carbohydrate, glucose which removes tiredness and weakness of body.

Day 8: In order to get accustomed to normal diet, partially normal food is introduced.

Guggulutikta kashaya
- 20 ml of decoction with 20 ml water before breakfast and dinner

Varasanadi Kashaya
- 20 ml of decoction with 20 ml water before breakfast and dinner

Varanadi Kashaya
- 20 ml of decoction with 20 ml water before breakfast and dinner

Navaka Guggulu
- 2 tablets after breakfast and dinner

Ayaskrti
- 20 ml of decoction with 20 ml water before breakfast and dinner

Asanadi Kashaya
- 20 ml of decoction with 20 ml water before breakfast and dinner

Mind – please take care!!

- Mind is most important factor for health and wellbeing.
- When mind is disturbed, eventually social relations are affected.
- Unless and until the mind is strong, no medicine would show its action completely.
- In the present life individuals are very sensitive and mentally weak, not even able to tackle even the minor problems.
- A strong mind can definitely manage the severe diseases, whereas a weak mind will not even be able to control smallest health condition.
- Ayurveda gives utmost importance in curing the diseases as well as managing the stressful daily life.

- Every person should concentrate on balancing, stabilizing and strengthening the mind instead of running behind the trend.
- A person should start a healthy and timely schedule.
- Practices like Meditation, Yoga, and Pranayama regularly helps in maintaining the balance of mind.

Spirituality

- Spirituality is the way of positive healthy living.
- Spirituality does not mean being religious.

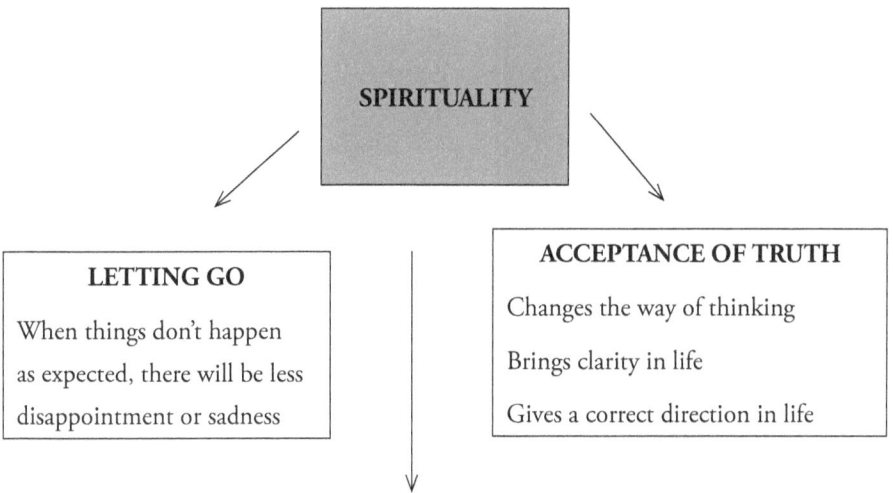

Chanting few sacred hymns (mantras) will help in bringing positivity, making the mind stable and calm.

Significance of chanting Om

- Om is the sound of creation and supreme power.
- By chanting Om, there will be increased oxygen to the body.
- Om purifies both body and mind.
- Chanting Om will remove all the obstacles in life.
- Chanting Om gives good immunity, self-healing and vibrations produced during the chanting opens up the blocked sinuses.
- One should sit in erect position, peaceful environment closing eyes and chant Om for 3–5 minutes.

Mrityunjaya Mantra (Victory over death/misfortunes)

"Om Trayambakam Yajaamahe

Sugandhim Pushtti Vardhanam

Urvaarukamiva Bandhanaan

Mrtyor Mukssiiya Maamrtaat"

Meaning of the Mantra

- Trayambaka means concentrating on the third eye which symbolizes the mind.
- Yajamahe means praying.
- The second line means this mantra gives us happiness, satisfaction, peace in life.
- The third and fourth combinely means avoiding untimely deaths, misfortunes.
- It helps to increase life span by chanting regularly.
- The best time to chant mantra is early in the morning and before going to work, before driving, before taking medicines or before sleep.

Gayatri Mantra

"Om bhur bhuvaswaha
Tatsa vithur varenyam
Bhargo devasyadhimahi
Dhiyoyonah prachodayath"

Meaning of the Mantra

- Om means Almighty God,
- Bhuh is the expression of vital, spiritual energy.
- Bhuvah is the destroyer of sufferings.
- Swah is the existence of happiness.
- Savituh which is bright shining object like sun.
- Varenyam means the best.
- Bhargo is the destroyer of sins.
- Devasya means which is divine.
- Dhimahi means imbibing.
- Dhiyo means intelligent.
- Yo means who.
- Nah means ours.
- Prachodayath means which is inspiring.

Benefits

- The mantra calms the mind, improves immunity.
- It increases concentration power, learning skills.
- It strengthens the nerves and heart.

- It also improves breathing, reduces stress and stress related body damage.
- The mantra brings positivity, development

One should chant the mantra 3 or 108 times for best results.

POSTURE RELATED PROBLEMS

- Different occupation has different types of posture.
- IT profession, telecaller jobs, coorporates, drivers, etc. will have to work on computers, speak on phones for long time.
- Hence they will have to adopt certain postures like bending the back, bending the neck, which would hamper the normal curvature or alignment of spine.
- It results in stiffness in the regions of neck, chest, hip and back.
- It also leads to numbness, pain in neck radiating to hands.
- It also leads to pain in the hip region or radiating to leg.
- Pain in calf muscles and foot is also another sign of improper posture.

Management

- First and foremost the posture is to be corrected

Chair

- Sit erect in a medium soft chair.
- Choose chair which has a straight back slight curved outwards at the middle.
- The chair should neither be too hard or nor too soft.
- Keep giving movements to the joints.

Yoga and exercise

- Regular yoga and exercise also helps to get rid of posture related problems.
- Yogasanas like Suryanamskara (sun salutation), *Vrikshasana, Bhujangasana* (cobra pose), *Shalabahsana* (locust pose), *Setubhandhasana, Shavasana* (corpse pose).
- Push ups, pull ups for a little duration also strengthens the muscles of arms, shoulders, chest.

Bed and sleep posture

- Sleeping with a pillow, which is neither too low nor too high.
- Sleeping in mattress which is comfortable and of even height.
- Always sleep in left lateral or right lateral position.
- It is better to avoid sleeping in prone or uneven posture as it affects the spine.

Ayurveda therapies for posture related disorders

Oil massage followed by steam with tube.

Oil like *Prabhanjana vimardana taila, Masha taila.*

- *Greeva vasti.*
- *Kati vasti.*
- *Pizhicil.*
- *Sarvanga kashayadhara* or *ksheera dhara.*

Pouch massage called *Naranga kizhi* or *Ela kizhi.*

Refer Fig 3.8

CLIMATE RELATED BODY PROBLEMS

In Extremely cold climatic conditions,

Commonly people will have problems like,

- Dry skin and hairs, cracked lips
- Muscle cramps
- Poor digestion
- Increased sleepiness
- Drop in body temperature, due to hampered of blood circulation
- Cold and fever
- Sore throat
- Asthma
- Headaches
- Swelling and inflamed joints

Diet

- Food and food types or drinks explained in Seasonal regimen for extreme winter are to be followed.
- Hot soups, hot beverages, food with spices like ginger, garlic, pepper, onion must be used.
- Soups like mixed vegetable, appetizer soup with extra spices can be taken.
- Food with adequate fats like ghee, butter, oil (moderate) quantity should be taken as it helps to correct digestion and provides moisture to skin.

Body care

- Application of oil to hairs, face and body must be done followed by hot water bath.

- Cover the head including ears and neck with thick or woolen clothes; also cover body with thick or woolen cloth.
- Remain in a warm chamber or near the fire place.

Activities
- Activities should be preferred indoor like yoga, crunches, pushups, squats etc.
- Activities and workouts can be done with full strength as person will have good energy.

Avoid
- Avoid fried, baked, dry food like toast, bread, cakes, and pastries.
- Dry fruits or nuts can be eaten in very little quantity.
- Avoid cold, chilled, tinned, packed food stuffs.
- One should never expose to external environment without covering your body with thick cloths or avoid going out at night.

Ayurveda procedures like
- Oil massage and head massage with *Brihat saindhavadi taila, Karpooradi taila, Marichadi taila* keeps the body warm.
- Whole body steam helps in loosening the stiff joints, reduce muscle cramps, regulates the dropped body temperature and enhances blood circulation.
- For exfoliation and as a fat burner or to keep the body warm, powder massage can be done using *Triphala choorna, Kola kulathadi choorna* (only after oil massage).
- *Kati vasti and Janu vasti* – these helps to reduce joint stiffness due to cold climate and helps to lubricate joints, reduces pain, reduces the degeneration of tissues.
- Face pack which is honey based or milk/milk cream based is advised here.

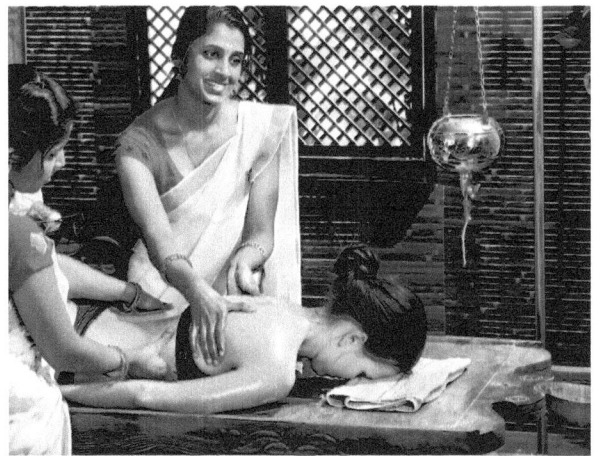

Fig 1.7 Oil Massage

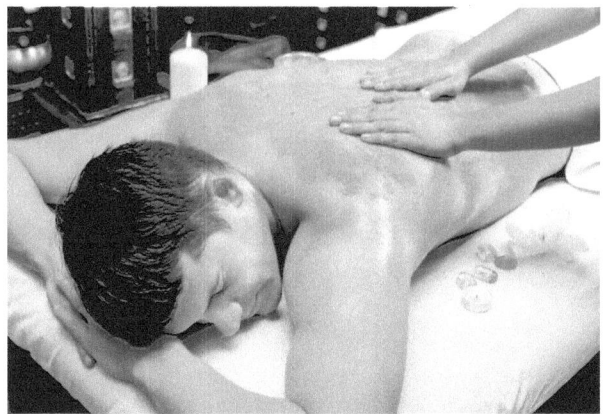

Fig 1.8 Powder Massage

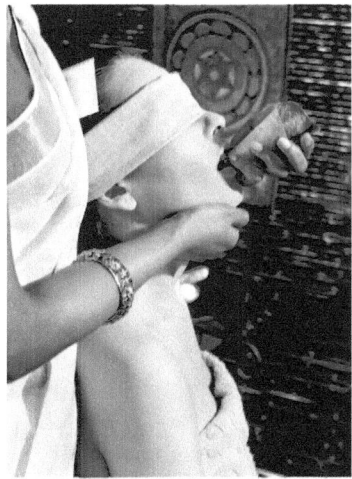

Fig 1.9 Snehapana

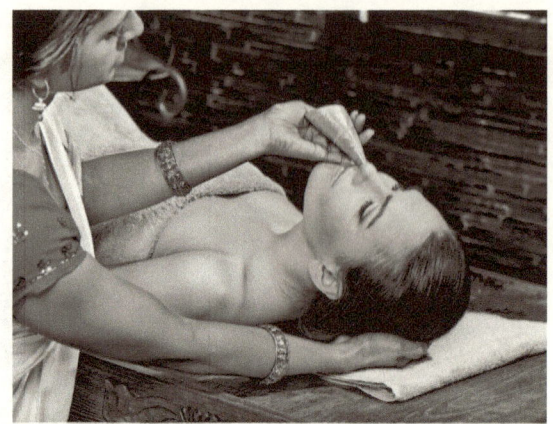

Fig 2.0 Nasya

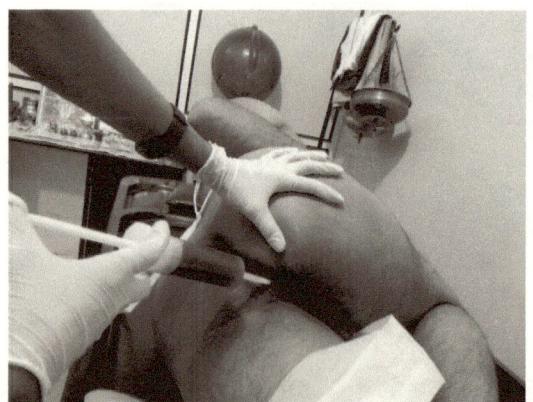

Fig 2.1 Vasthi

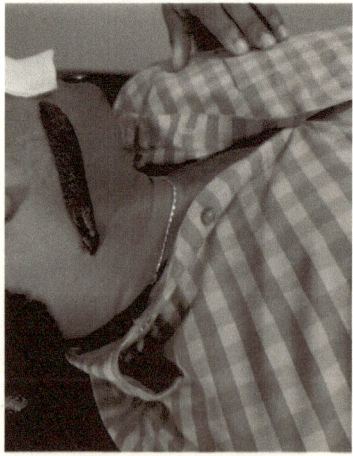

Fig 2.2 Raktamokshana

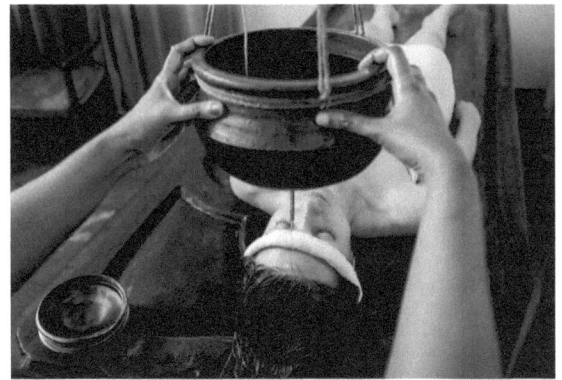

Fig 2.3 Shirodhara

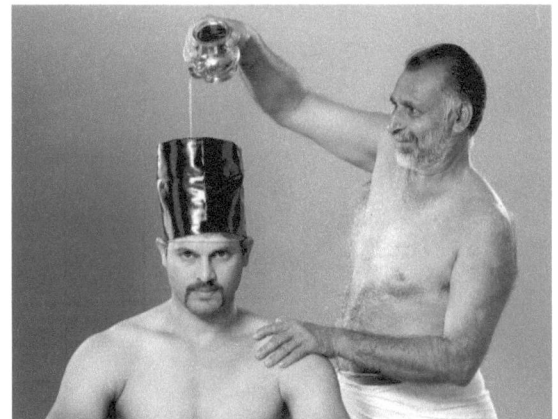

Fig 2.4 Shirovasti

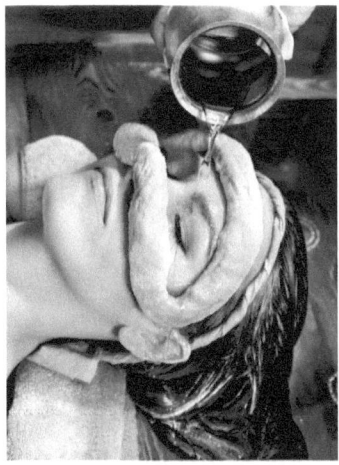

Fig 2.5 Netra Tarpana

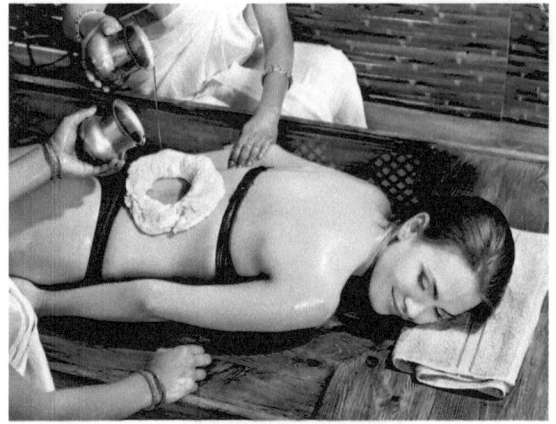

Fig 2.6 Kati Vasti

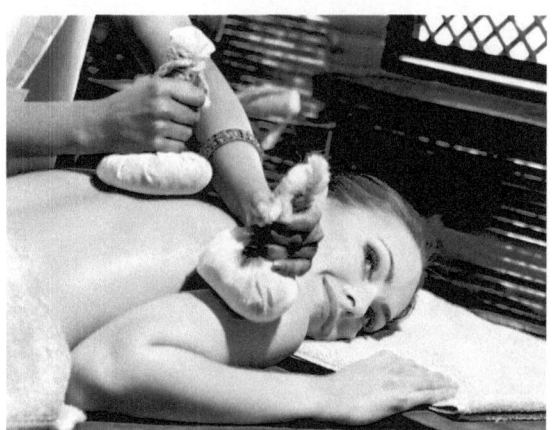

Fig 2.7 Ela Kizhi

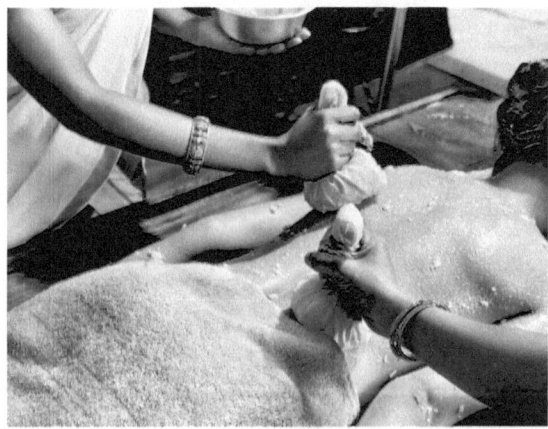

Fig 2.8 Njavarkizhi

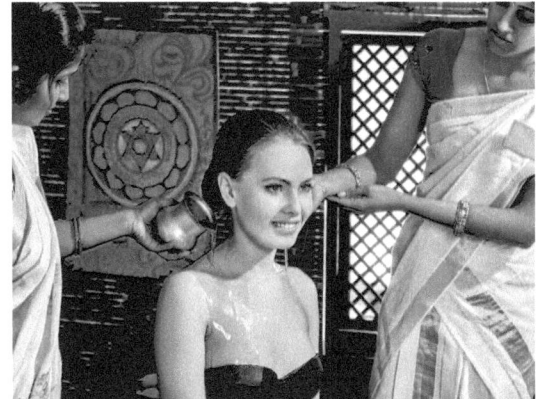

Fig 2.9 Pizhichil

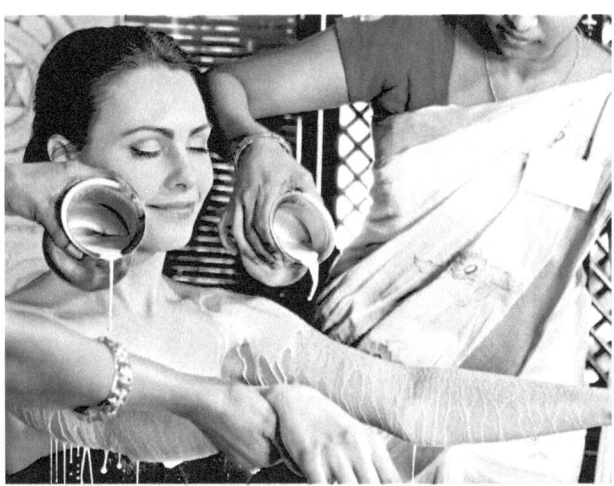

Fig 3.0 Saravanga Kashayaksira Dhara

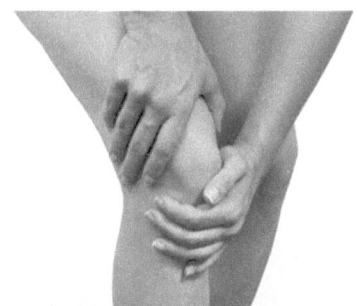

Fig 3.1 Rhematoid Arthrittis

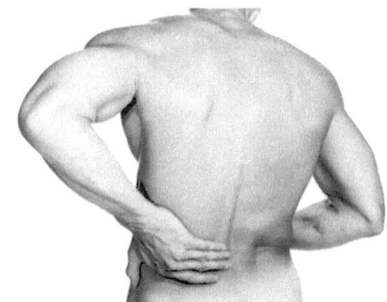

Fig 3.2 Low Back Pain

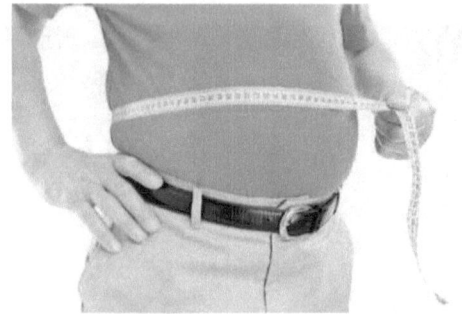

Fig 3.3 Obesity

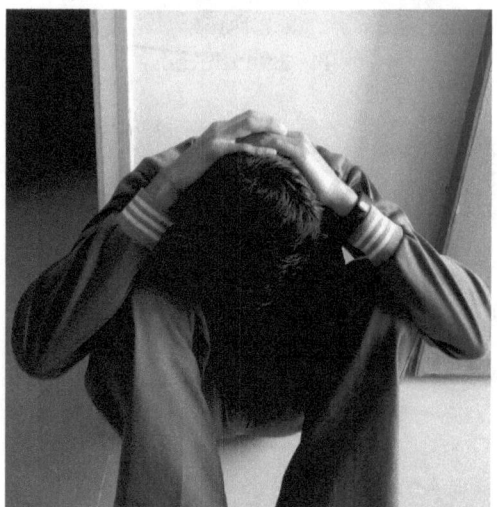

Fig 3.4 Depression

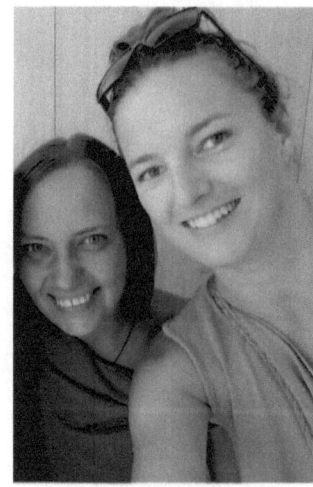

Fig 3.5 Skin Care

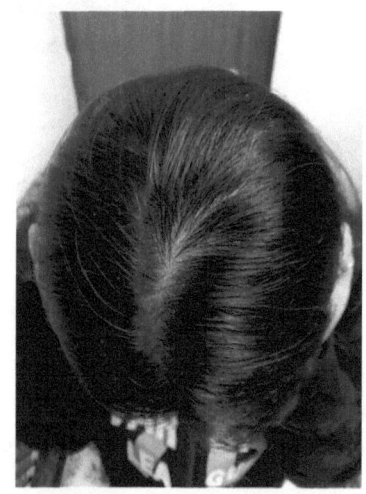

Fig 3.6 Hair Care

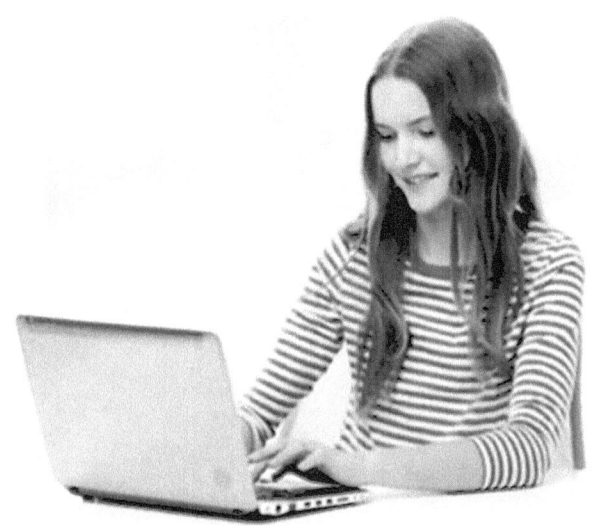
Fig 3.7 Occupational Care

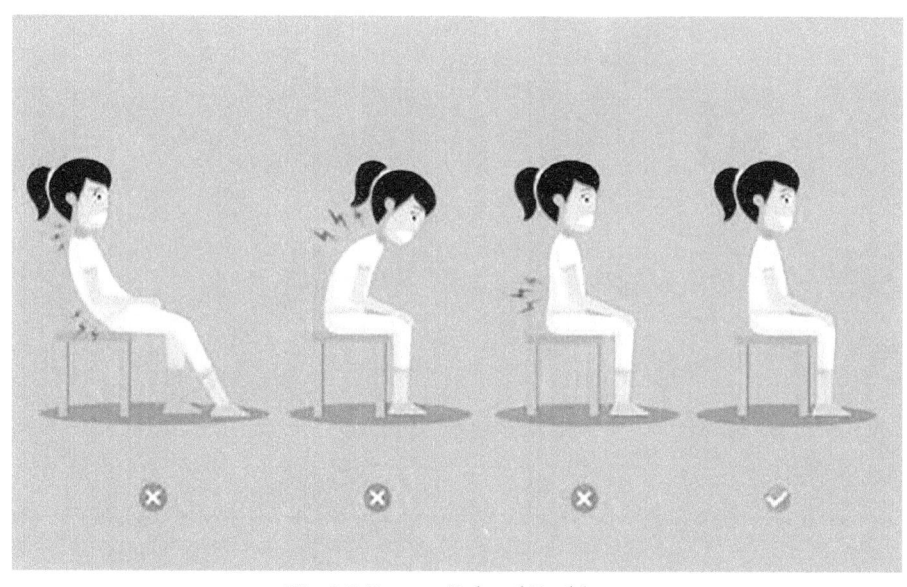
Fig 3.8 Posture Related Problems

CONCEPTS OF FOOD

- KITCHEN CONCEPTS — 243
- LIQUID FOOD — 245
- MEDICATED WATER — 246
- GINGER WATER — 246
- CUMIN SEED WATER — 246
- BASIL LEAF WATER — 246
- CINNAMON WATER — 247

CONCEPTS OF FOOD

KITCHEN CONCEPTS

- Kitchen is an integral part of every house from where the health begins.
- Diet when followed wrong, gives rise to most of the diseases.
- The kitchen is ideally to be located facing South-east or at least North-east.
- There are many things to be taken care about the kitchen one out of which is hygiene.
- Right Equipments used in kitchen contributes to health and tasty food.
- Utensils used in the kitchen have its own impact on adding nutrition to the food.

Gold utensil: it makes the body strong by boosting immunity.

Silver utensil: it cools down the body and helps to improve vision.

Bronze utensil: it improves the appetite, purifies blood and increases intellect.

Never eat any sour substance in this vessel as it may react and cause toxic affect.

Copper utensil: water is to be stored in this utensil as it purifies the blood. Improves the memory power and removes toxins from the body.

Milk products should never be consumed in this vessel as it may react and turn toxic.

Brass utensil: it is extensively used in feeding children as it destroys worms from the body. It imparts strength to the body.

Iron utensil: it gives good iron supplement to the body making it strong enough.

Milk drunk using iron vessel can increase the memory power.

Aluminium utensil: it should never be sued in cooking as it destroys almost half of the nutrients present in food.

But unfortunately most of the pressure cookers are made up of aluminium.

Steel utensil: it doesn't react with any kind of food materials nor provides benefits to the body.

Earthen utensil: food cooked in the vessel gives maximum nutrients and cools down the body. It imparts very good taste to the food prepared in it.

It is very economical but should be cooked with care.

Teflon coated or Nonstick utensil: most of the people used it as it makes cooking very easy and less messy. But it has its own worst effect on the body.

- When the food is cooked in this it causes toxins in the body and may cause Cancer.
- One should recite the mantra before eating food.

"*Sahana Vavatu Sahanau Bunnattu Sahaveeryam Karavavahai*

Tejasvina Vadhi Tamastu Ma Vidhvishavahai"

Let God protect us

Let he nourish me and my mind.

May God give us the energy.

May our knowledge be sharp and effective

May we mutually not dispute.

Concepts of Food

- While listening to the word Ayurveda, first thing what strikes in peoples mind is herbs, salads etc., and of course "Vegetarian diet."
- The truth is, Ayurveda believes in balanced diet.
- A person who is healthy should always prefer balanced diet rather being than a pure vegetarian or a pure non-vegetarian.
- A healthy diet should contain vegetables, fruits, meat, fish, egg in a moderate quantity and which is processed in a good and systematic way.
- One can include more of vegetables and fruits in your diet but non vegetarian should be included 2–3 times a week.
- Breakfast should include food which is light and easily digestible
- One has food like idly, dosa, juice, boiled egg, milk, pancakes.
- If one eats heavy, fried, baked food in the morning then you would feel very heavy, uncomfortable and drowsy all day.

Types of food or forms of food

LIQUID FOOD

- Liquid food is always the lightest form of food. But few can be heavier example: yogurt.
- We usually give liquid for the person with weak digestive power as carminative or digestive.

MEDICATED WATER

General Method of Preparation
- Herbs: 30 gms
- Water: 500 ml
- Mix the herbs in the water and boil it till it reduces to half the quantity (250 ml). Filter it and consume it hot or warm.

GINGER WATER

- Ginger water is a good appetizer, corrects digestion, enhances taste buds, and relieves the bloating of abdomen.
- Ginger can be given in Common cold, Cough, Constipation, Arthritis, and Obesity.

Refer Fig 3.9

CUMIN SEED WATER

- Cumin seed water corrects the digestion, metabolism, eliminates the gas troubles in body.
- It can be given for Acidity, pain in the abdomen, Fever, Dysmenorrhea.

BASIL LEAF WATER

- It increases the immunity in body towards Cold, Cough, Viral fever, Sinusitis.

CINNAMON WATER

- It increases the digestion, corrects the fat metabolism and removes bad odor from mouth.
- It is effective in Obesity, Diabetes, high cholesterol, Arthritis.

FRESH JUICES

- METHOD OF PREPARATION — 251
- LEMON JUICE — 251
- GRAPE JUICE — 251
- POMEGRANATE JUICE — 252
- ORANGE JUICE — 252
- WATERMELON JUICE — 252
- PAPAYA JUICE — 252
- MANGO JUICE — 252
- CRANBERRY JUICE — 253
- AVOCADO JUICE — 253
- CARROT JUICE — 253

FRESH JUICES

METHOD OF PREPARATION

- Juices should be fresh, avoid refrigerating it.
- Take fruits like apple, grape, papaya, watermelon, orange, etc.
- Remove the seeds, cut into medium pieces.
- Grind it in mixer with sufficient water and sugar.
- Carrot should be slightly cooked first then blended in mixer, add little water, and is ready to drink.
- Never add milk and always use moderate quantity of sugar.

LEMON JUICE

- It enhances taste, increase digestion, and subsides nausea,
- It helps in reducing the excessive heat in body, and gaining strength when added with honey, jaggery, and sugar candy.

GRAPE JUICE

- It enhances taste, improves the absorption of essential nutrients in the body and relieves constipation.
- It is beneficial in increasing the blood count, and it is a cardiac tonic.

POMEGRANATE JUICE

- It improves taste perception, enhances digestion, and helps in relieving acidity as well as constipation.
- It increases hemoglobin of blood, enhances skin texture- quality- complexion.

ORANGE JUICE

- It increases digestion of food, enhances skin quality - complexion.
- It also improves eye sight.

WATERMELON JUICE

- It cools the body, helps in rehydrating the body especially in summer season.
- It is the best supplement of sugar/glucose- sodium-potassium.

PAPAYA JUICE

- It helps in relieving constipation; platelet count is increased by taking the juice of its leaf especially in fever like Dengue.
- It is also good for skin and liver diseases.

MANGO JUICE

- It enhances taste perception.
- It provides energy in terms of nutrition in summer season.

CRANBERRY JUICE

- It is good anti-oxidant; it enhances the functions of blood.
- It is also good for heart.

AVOCADO JUICE

- It is good anti-oxidant, good to control hypertension, cholesterol levels and also a skin texture enhancer.

CARROT JUICE

- It improves appetite, digestion, eye sight, improves eyesight, and enhances skin texture.

MEDICINAL JUICES

- AMLA JUICE 257
- ALOE VERA JUICE 257
- COCUM JUICE 257
- INDIAN MULBERRY JUICE 257
- SARSAPARILLA JUICE 258
- VETIVER ROOT JUICE 258
- BITTER GOURD JUICE 258
- BLACK PLUM JUICE (JAMUN) 258

MEDICINAL JUICES

AMLA JUICE

- It is best anti-oxidant, good for hair growth, improves eyesight.
- It controls Diabetes, is Vitamin C source and best rejuvenative juice.

Refer Fig 4.0

ALOE VERA JUICE

- It helps to reduce acidity, a very good liver tonic, corrects delayed and scanty menstrual flow, and controls blood sugar level.

COCUM JUICE

- Cocum juice is sour, which helps to reduce body fat, reduces acidity.
- It reduces thirst especially in summer, brings down cholesterol levels.

Refer Fig 4.1

INDIAN MULBERRY JUICE

- It is good antioxidant, builds up the immune system of body, and has anti cancerous property.

SARSAPARILLA JUICE

- It is a coolant, relieves acidity, body heat, and purifies the skin.

VETIVER ROOT JUICE

- It is a coolant, reduces body heat, maintains blood pressure, and purifies skin.

BITTER GOURD JUICE

- It stimulates the liver cells, and maintains blood sugar level.

BLACK PLUM JUICE (JAMUN)

- It is useful in Diarrhea; it cools down the body and is effective for Diabetic patients.

MILK AND MILK PRODUCTS

- FIVE COW PRODUCTS 261
- MILK AND MILK PRODUCTS 261
- COW'S PRODUCT 262

MILK AND MILK PRODUCTS

FIVE COW PRODUCTS

- Milk
- Yogurt
- Ghee
- Cows Urine
- Cow Dung

MILK AND MILK PRODUCTS

Milk (cow's milk): It is very good rejuvenative, best calcium supplement and good for bones.

It is effective in Insomnia, increases sperm count in men, as well as lactation in women.

Yoghurt: Yoghurt increases the protein, calcium in body, sperm count as well as body weight.

Buttermilk: Buttermilk increases appetite, digestion as well as metabolism.

It relieves Constipation, Hemorrhoid, Acidity, cures tastelessness, Anemia.

Butter: It is a coolant.

It builds the body by nourishing it, cures hemorrhoids, and relieves throat irritation.

Ghee: Ghee is an anti-oxidant, increases digestive fire.

It builds up vitality, intellect, memory, vision, color, and complexion, sweetness of voice.

It is the best rejuvenative.

Cheese: Cheese is heavy for digestion, yet nourishing and muscle bulk promoter.

But it needs to be carefully consumed as it may cause indigestion.

If taken too much leads to increased cholesterol and body fat.

COW'S PRODUCT

- 5 products obtained from Cow namely milk, yogurt, ghee, cow's urine and cow dung.
- Milk, yogurt and ghee properties are as explained above.

Cow's urine: It can be used alone or as a mixture with other herbs in diseases like skin, cancer, anemia, epilepsy.

It also has remarkable property to reduce body fat and reduced cholesterol levels.

It is said to have antifungal and also antimicrobial.

Thus it is sprinkled in places around the house or where people reside.

But people with increased or diseases of *Pitha dosha* vitiation, should take it with cautiousness as it would worsen the condition.

Cow dung: It is best used as manure and used as mosquito repellent when mixed with herbs.

- It is not really used for internal medicine.
- A special ghee is prepared where all five products from cow are used.
- It is effective in epilepsy, psychosis or mental disorders and this ghee is indicated in improving brain functions.

SOUPS

- RICE WATER SOUP   267
- CARROT SOUP   268
- BEETROOT SOUP   268
- TOMATO SOUP   269
- SPINACH SOUP   270
- MIXED VEGETABLE SOUP   272

SOUPS

RICE WATER SOUP

Ingredients

- Brown rice 200 gms
- Water 600 ml
- Salt to taste

Method of preparation

- Keep water for boiling in a vessel.
- Once the water starts boiling add the washed rice and cook until done.
  1. Take 1 tbsp.of rice and grind it into a paste.
  2. Add with 1 glass of rice water to it.
  3. Add salt.

Benefits

- It is very light, best for indigestion, helps in electrolyte balance, and relieves tiredness.
- It is specially given after detoxification therapy as it supports and strengthens digestive system.

CARROT SOUP

Ingredients

- Carrot 4 medium sized
- Garlic 3 cloves
- Ginger 1 inch
- Onion 1 large, diced
- Pepper to taste
- Salt to taste

Method of preparation

1. The cleaned carrot should be kept in pressure cooker until 2–3 whistles.
2. In a pan, add 2 tsp. of oil; add onion and garlic.
   - Cook it till onion becomes translucent.
3. Add cooked carrot and ginger stir it for 3–4 min.
4. Heat this puree just before serving.

Soup is ready

Benefits

- Same as that of carrot juice but more digestive and appetizer.

BEETROOT SOUP

Ingredients

- Beetroots 2
- Onion 1 (chopped)
- Tomato 2 (cut)

- Garlic 3–4 cloves
- Pepper corns 5–6
- Cinnamon 1 inch
- Water 350 ml
- Coconut oil 2 tbsp.

Method of preparation

1. Heat the oil in a pan and add pepper, cinnamon and garlic, sauté lightly till the smell appears.
2. Add chopped onions sauté it up till golden brown color.
3. Tomato should be added and to be tossed continuously, until the tomato skin wrinkles.
4. Add beetroot, salt and water.
    - Keep it in pressure cook until 2–3 whistles appears.
5. Blend it into smooth puree using mixer or blender.
6. Add the soup to a pan and continue until a small boil appears and simmer it for 3–4 min.

Ready to serve

Benefits

- It is good for skin; improve its texture and color.
- It is also good for digestive system as it is fibrous.
- It purifies the blood and enhances circulatory system.

TOMATO SOUP

Ingredients

- Garlic 3–4 clove
- Peppercorns 7–8

- Bay leaf small
- Butter ½ tbsp.
- Sugar 1 tsp.
- Water 1 ½ cup
- Salt to taste

Method of preparation

1. Cut tomatoes into big pieces.
2. Add cut tomatoes, pepper corns, garlic and bay leaf in pressure cooker with 1 cup of water and salt. Cook for 2–3 whistles.
3. Let the mixture be cool and then put it into blender/mixer.
    - Make smooth puree (remove the bay leaf).
4. Strain it using sieve, throw away the residue.
5. In a deep bottom pan heat butter, add strained tomato pure, add sugar and boil it.
6. Add water if required, cook it for 6–7 min.
7. Garnish with pepper powder and coriander leaves.

Benefits

- It is a taste enhancer and a good appetizer.
- It is the best source of vitamin C, hence good for skin and eyes.

Refer Fig 4.2

SPINACH SOUP

Ingredients

- Spinach 2 cups
- Onion chopped 1 big
- Tomato chopped 1 medium

- Green chili 1 small
- Ginger ¼ inch
- Garlic 2 cloves
- Water 1 ½ cup
- Ghee 1 tsp.
- Garlic paste 1 tsp.
- Pepper powder ¼ tsp.
- Salt to taste

Method of preparation

1. Take a deep bottom pan, add little butter and roast onion, green chili, ginger and garlic.
2. Add water to it and boil on medium flame for 10–12 minutes.
3. Add washed leaves of spinach, cook it for 3–4 min.
4. Turn of the flame and allow it to cool for 3–4 min.
5. Put it into mixer and make a smooth puree of it.
6. Heat butter in a pan, add garlic paste.
   - Sauté for 1–2 min, and add the puree.
7. Add water as per you like (not to thin or thick).
8. Add salt and pepper, simmer for 5 min and bring it to boil. Turn off the gas

Spinach soup ready to taste

Benefits

- It is the best vitamin supplement, with fewer calories.
- It is iron rich, thus, supporting function of red blood cells and increase oxygen absorption capacity.
- It helps in maintaining the bone health as it provides calcium supplement to body.

Refer Fig 4.3

MIXED VEGETABLE SOUP

Ingredients

- Onion 1 (mediums sized, roughly chopped)
- Tomato 1 (big sized, roughly chopped)
- Capsicum 1 (medium sized roughly chopped)
- Cabbage ¼ cups
- Pepper ¼ tsp.
- Salt to taste

Method of preparation

1. In a pressure cooker add onions, roast till golden brown
2. Add tomatoes, capsicum, and cabbage for 3 min.
3. Add 1 ½ cups of water and mix well in pressure cook for 3–4 whistles.
4. Cool it after it is cooked, add into mixer jar and make a puree of it.
5. Transfer soup into deep pan; add pepper, salt.

Cook it on medium flame for 2 min.

Serve hot

Benefits

- Mixed vegetable soup contains more vitamins as it is mixture of vegetables.
- It is light for digestion.
- It is also best for cough, cold and constipation.

TEA

- HERBAL TEA — 275
- SPICES TEA — 276
- TULASI TEA — 277

TEA

HERBAL TEA

Ingredients
- Coriander seeds: 2 tbsp.
- Cumin seed: 1 tbsp.
- Fenugreek seed: 4–5
- Pepper corn: 5–6
- Cardamom: 4–5
- Cinnamon 2 inch stick.

Note: Take all the ingredients, dry it under the sun for 3–4 days. Slightly roast it and make it into coarse powder.

Method of preparation
- Take powder and other ingredients, boil in 500 ml water.
- Boil it properly, add jaggery and stir.
- Filter it and is ready for drinking.

Benefits
- Herbs in this recipe are one with hot potency, and little cold potency.
- Thus it helps to balance the blood circulation.
- It relives headache and keeps one fresh throughout the day.

- It also helps to relive bloating of abdomen, indigestion, cough, cold, and acts as appetizer.

SPICES TEA

Ingredients

- Tea powder or tea bags 3–4
- Cinnamon 1 small stick
- Cardamom 3–4
- Cloves 2–3
- Ginger 1 small piece
- Water 300 ml

Method of preparation

1. Take a sauce pan and boil water in it.
2. Add tea bags to it.
3. Add cinanmom sticks, cardamom, cloves and ginger piece and bring it to boil and simmer for 2–3 min.
4. Filter it, add milk and required quantity of sugar.

Benefits

- Tea along with these wonderful spices refreshes the taste buds, removes foul smell in the mouth.
- Hence it prevents oral diseases.
- It improves digestion, relives constipation and bloating of stomach.
- It also acts as slimming tea, as cinnamon and cloves are part of it.

TULASI TEA

Ingredients

- *Tulasi* leaves ¼ cup
- *Tulasi* stem 5–6
- Clove 1
- Cumin seeds ¼ spoons
- Peppercorns 1–2
- Water 4 cups
- Lemon ½ tsp.

Method of preparation

1. Dry roast pepper corn, cumin seeds and clove on pan and powder it coarsely in mortar pestle.
2. Chop *Tulasi* leaves finely and chop the stem of *Tulasi* too.
3. Mix the powdered spices, chopped leaves, *Tulasi* stem and pound it again in mortar pestle till becomes coarse.
4. Boil 4 cups of water and add coarsely ground ingredients and reduce it to half.

Filter the decoction and drink it warm.

Benefits

- *Tulasi* tea which has multiple actions as *Tulasi* is most potent herb.
- It can relieve cold, cough, fever, headache like symptoms.
- It also acts best in obese people and good for digestive disorders.
- It is best blood purifier keeping skin healthy and maintains oral hygiene.

Refer Fig 4.4

SALADS

- CAPSICUM ONION CARROT SALAD — 281
- CUCUMBER COCONUT SALAD — 281
- CARROT ONION SALAD — 282
- TOMATO ONION SALAD — 282
- CAPSICUM ONION CABBAGE SALAD — 283
- FRUIT SALAD — 283

SALADS

CAPSICUM ONION CARROT SALAD

Ingredients

- Capsicum 1 medium
- Onion sliced 1 big
- Carrot sliced 1 medium
- Pepper powder ¼ tsp.
- Salt to taste

Method of preparation

- Mix capsicum, onion and carrot and add salt and pepper powder, mix well.

CUCUMBER COCONUT SALAD

Ingredients

- Cucumber: 1 medium
- Coconut (grated): 1 cup
- Soaked green gram: half cup (overnight soaked)
- Pepper powder ¼ tsp.
- Curry leaves: 4–5 leaves
- Salt to taste

Method of preparation

- Chop the cucumber and onion into small pieces.
- Mix soaked green gram and pepper powder
- Splutter curry leaves in 1 tsp. of oil. Add to the above mixture.

CARROT ONION SALAD

Ingredients

- Carrot grated 1 medium
- Coconut (grated) 1 cup
- Onion 1 big
- Pepper powder ¼ tsp.
- Lemon juice 1 tsp.
- Salt to taste

Method of preparation

1. Take grated carrot and add chopped onion to it.
2. Add salt and pepper
3. Add coconut and lemon juice, mix well.

TOMATO ONION SALAD

Ingredients

- Onion 1 (big sized)
- Tomato 1 (medium sized)
- Pepper powder 1 pinch
- Salt to taste

Method of preparation

1. Chop onion and tomato into small pieces.
2. Take all the ingredients in a bowl, mix well.

CAPSICUM ONION CABBAGE SALAD

Ingredients

- Cabbage chopped 1 cup
- Onion sliced 1 big
- Pepper powder ¼ tsp.
- Salt to taste

Method of preparation

1. Mix well all the ingredients in a bowl

FRUIT SALAD

Ingredients

- Papaya 1 cup
- Banana ½ cup
- Apple ½ cup
- Pomegranate ½ cup
- Black salt 1 pinch
- Honey 1 tbsp.

Method of preparation

    1. All fruits are sliced into medium pieces and taken in a bowl.

    2. Black salt and honey is added into it and mixed well.

SANDWICH

- HEALTHY SANDWICH   287
- SPECIAL SANDWICH   288

SANDWICH

HEALTHY SANDWICH

Ingredients

- Bread 1 loaf small
- Onion round slices 10
- Cucumber round slices 10
- Tomato round slices 10
- Tomato sauce 4 tbsp.
- Coriander leaves 1 bunch
- Green chilies 2 small
- Garlic 4–5 clove

Method of preparation

1. Prepare the paste of coriander leaves, green chilies and garlic, add little salt to it.
2. Take 2 breads apply a little tomato sauce and apply 2 tsp. of coriander paste on both.
3. Keep the slices of onion, tomato, cucumber on one bread piece.
4. Cover it with other piece of bread and roast it slightly over pan.

Benefits

- It can be given to children in the breakfast or snacks as it nutritive.
- It is light for digestion.
- It is good for weight loss if eaten in less quantity.

SPECIAL SANDWICH

Ingredients

- Wheat bread (brown bread)
- Prepare Paste by grinding coriander leaves (1/2 bunch) with fenugreek leaves (10–12 leaves) along with ginger and garlic and salt

Method of preparation

- Paste is little different as fenugreek leaves are added

Benefits

- Wheat bread is more digestive and has fewer calories.
- It can be taken by people who are eager to lose weight or shed few pounds.

SAUCE

- BANANA (NENDRA) SAUCE — 291
- MANGO SAUCE — 292
- SALTED MANGO SAUCE — 292
- CORIANDER TAMARIND SAUCE — 293
- ONION SAUCE — 293
- BENEFITS OF ALL SAUCES — 294

SAUCE

- Sauces are tasty, can be consumed in breakfast or lunch with chapatti, rice, pancakes.
- It is light for digestion and good appetizer.
- Sauces of fruits are best for nutrition.
- When it is taken with bread, it removes the dry property of bread and is easy for digestion.

BANANA (NENDRA) SAUCE

Ingredients

- Banana 2 big
- Pepper corns 6–7
- Water ¾ cup
- Ghee 2 tsp.
- Jaggery 2 tsp.

Method of preparation

1. Remove the skin of big banana, cut it into small pieces.
2. Smash jaggery, pepper corns and salt.
3. Add water to above mixture.
4. Add the banana pieces and smash with hands.
5. Heat the ghee in small pan.

Add curry leaves and splutter, add to above mixture.

MANGO SAUCE

Ingredients

- Mango 1 big
- Peppercorns 6–7
- Water ¾ cup
- Ghee 2 tsp.
- Jaggery 2 tsp.

Method of preparation

1. Remove the skin of big mango, cut it into small pieces and mash it.
2. Smash jaggery, pepper corns and salt.
3. Add water to above mixture.
4. Add the mashed mango and press with hands.
5. Heat the ghee in small pan, add curry leaves and splutter, add to above mixture.

SALTED MANGO SAUCE

Ingredients

- Salted mango 1 big
- Pepper corns 10
- Water ½ cup
- Oil 2 spoon
- Pea sized asafetida in 2 tsp. of water

Method of preparation

1. Powder the pepper corns, smash salted mango with ½ cup of water.
2. Add 2 tsp. of oil and asafetida water.

CORIANDER TAMARIND SAUCE

Ingredients

- Coriander leaves one bunch
- Tamarind lemon sized
- Jaggery small orange sized
- Pepper corns 6–7
- Salt

Method of preparation

1. Wash coriander leaves
2. Grind tamarind, jaggery, salt, pepper corns, coriander leaves in mixer into fine paste (add little water).

Tamarind sauce ready to taste.

ONION SAUCE

Ingredients

- Onion 3–4 medium size
- Red chili flakes ½ tsp.
- Tamarind pea sized

- Oil 2 tsp.
- Water ½ cup
- Salt for taste

Method of preparation

1. Take pepper powder, tamarind and salt and smash with smasher adding water.
2. To above mixtures add finely chopped onion, and add oil.

Onion sauce ready to taste.

BENEFITS OF ALL SAUCES

- Sauces are highly digestive in nature.
- Sauces can be consumed even in rainy and winter season.
- It has less calories and suitable for all body types.

SPECIAL LIGHT FOOD

- OATS (WHOLE GRAIN)   297
- MUESLI OATS   297
- CORN FLAKES   297
- GRANOLA   298
- PASTA   298
- INDIAN WHEAT BREAD   299
- IDLY   300

SPECIAL LIGHT FOOD

OATS (WHOLE GRAIN)

- The form oats itself is light, so it can be taken (basically) in the night.
- It can be cooked simply with water to make it lighter.
- When it is cooked with milk, sugar and little dry fruits it is more nourishing.
- It is healthy for regular bowel movements.

MUESLI OATS

- Muesli oats is a mixture of dry fruits, fruits, milk and little of sweetening agents.
- It is tasty as well as healthy.
- It nourishes the body.
- Muesli oats can be more effective in people who are lean, tired and who have disturbed sleep.

CORN FLAKES

- Corn flakes are lighter and dry in nature.
- Corn flakes when cooked with milk and sweet substance (like sugar candy, jaggery) becomes healthy and softens the bowel.

- It is better to avoid in persons with Constipation and reduced bowel movements.
- It should also be avoided by people with dry skin, thin body (usually in people who has difficulty to gain weight).

GRANOLA

- Granola is composed of oats, nuts, honey, puffed rice which is baked.
- It is combined and eaten with yogurt, honey, and banana.
- Granola is rich in vitamins, minerals, fibrous, iron, and very much nutritive.
- It lowers the bad cholesterol; it is easy for digestion, increases energy.
- It lowers blood pressure, builds stronger bones, and increases body weight.
- It is good for people with dry skin, lean body, loss of energy.

PASTA

- Pasta is made of flour from cereals (buck wheat, quinoa, and chia) and grains (wheat, rice).
- It is healthy source of carbohydrates, when prepared in a healthy manner would yield best nutritive values.
- It should be cooked with very less oil and fresh vegetables.
- Pasta can be consumed by people with good digestive fire and power.
- It may lead to digestive problems in people with impaired digestive fire.

INDIAN WHEAT BREAD

Ingredients

- Wheat flour 1cup (250 gms)
- Water (warm)/Milk 50 ml (sufficient to make dough that doesn't stick to hand and can be rolled)
- Oil 2 tsp. (optional)
- Salt for taste

Method of preparation

- Wheat flour is made into dough using water or milk with or without oil.
- Then it is rolled into circular flat shape using roller.
- It is then roasted over fire by flipping it one side other.
- It can be directly kept over fire and flipped without oil. If needed one can add oil.
- This form of wheat bread becomes light to digest.

Benefits

- It can be consumed in conditions like Obesity, Diabetes where *Kapha dosha* is disturbed.
- It strengthens the body, helps in quick reunion of fractured bone.
- It also helps in degeneration of tissue/bones (when prepared adding oil/ghee).

Refer Fig 4.5

IDLY

Ingredients

- ½ cup black gram
- 1 tbsp.enugreek seeds
- 2 cups parboiled rice
- 1 cup long grain rice or any rice
- ¼ cup flattened or beaten rice
- Salt to taste

Method of preparation

1. Wash black gram and fenugreek seeds and soak it together with flattened rice for 4–5 hours.
2. Wash also parboiled rice and long grain rice and soak in water for 3–4 hours.
3. Drain water from soaked black gram and don't discard the water as it can be used during grinding.
4. Transfer the black gram and fenugreek seeds in large jar mixer or wet grinder, add 1/2cup of above water gradually until smooth and fluffy texture is achieved. The batter should neither be thin not thick.
5. Drain excess water from rice. Add drained rice in same mixer or wet grinder.
6. Add water in little amount (1/2 cup) and grind until coarse paste obtained.
7. Mix both black gram and rice paste in same container (the container has to be big).
8. Add salt to taste and mix well. If batter is thick idly turns hard and turn flat if too thin batter.

9. Place it in room temperature. But in the winter place in warm place. As cool atmosphere slows down fermentation for 8–10 hours.
10. Stir the batter the next day and place it in steamer with closed lid and cook for 10 min.

Check whether the Idlis are cooked, by inserting a knife or toothpick in center of idly, if it comes out clean then Idlis are cooked well, if not steam for few more minutes.

Serve with coconut sauce or Sāmbhar.

Benefits

- Idly is mainly made up of black gram and white rice.
- Both ingredients are taken in certain proportions and grinded.
- This is kept for a day, and allowed for fermentation.
- Next day it is cooked in steamer.
- Usually black gram is very heavy; as this is steamed the heavy quality turns lighter.
- Idly is strength promoter, nourishes body, can be taken by a person with *Vata* dosha and lean body structure.
- It is good for vitality and acts as aphrodisiac.

To be avoided in below conditions

- Yet, this should be avoided in conditions like indigestion, skin diseases,
- Especially in *Pitha* (skin eruptions, Eczema, hyperacidity) and *Kapha* diseases it should be avoided as it may worsen the condition.

Refer Fig 4.6

PANCAKE

- RICE PANCAKE — 305
- RED LENTIL PANCAKE — 306
- BROWN RICE PANCAKE — 307
- GHEE ROAST PANCAKE — 308
- ONION PANCAKE — 309
- CUCUMBER PANCAKE (SWEET AND SPICY) — 311
- SPICY CUCUMBER PANCAKE — 312
- SPICY PANCAKE — 312

PANCAKE

RICE PANCAKE

Ingredients

- Regular rice 1 cup
- Water 1.5 cup
- Coconut 1 tbsp.
- Salt for taste
- Oil for dosa

Method of preparation

1. Soak 1cup of rice in water till it dips in it for 5–10 hours (or overnight).
2. Drain the soaked rice put it into mixer along with coconut and add enough water to make a smooth paste.
3. Transfer it into other bowl and add enough water to make it flowing water consistency.
4. Add salt to taste and stir well.
5. Heat pan and take batter in a ladle (full).
6. Pour it on the hot pan and spread it completely to cover the whole pan.
7. Cover it with lid to cook (1 min) and then fold it into triangle
8. Water dosa ready.

This pancake is made using white rice and with or without coconut.

Benefits

- This is very light, very much digestive, and used in a weight loss diet.
- Can be taken even during indigestion as it is light and good taste.
- This should be taken with honey as it hastens weight loss.

Refer Fig 4.7

RED LENTIL PANCAKE

Ingredients

- Red lentil 100 gms
- Raw white rice 250 gms
- Water (to make batter)
- Salt to taste
- Coconut 2 tbsp.(optional)
- Garlic 2–3 pods
- Cumin ½ tsp.

Method of preparation

- Soak the red lentils and rice for about 5–6 hours or overnight.
- Grind it into smooth paste with quantity sufficient water to make it batter of medium consistency.
- Add coconut while grinding
- Add pieces of garlic and cumin seeds to the batter
- Heat the pan and smear little oil, take a ladle and mix it well. Take ladle full of batter and pour it over pan and spread it using back of ladle into round shape.

- Cover it for 1 min, add little oil and roast it according to your choice.
- Ready to eat red lentil pancake.

Benefits

- Red lentil pancake is specially prepared with garlic, cumin.
- It is has much of protein and fiber content.
- It aggravates *Vata dosha* as it is dry but garlic and cumin along with it would avoid the imbalance of *Vata dosha*.

To be avoided in:

- Person with increased body stiffness, cramping of muscles, problems of bone and spine, Osteo arthritis, lean body structure as more of light and dry quality

BROWN RICE PANCAKE

Ingredients

- Brown rice 100 gm
- White rice 100 gm
- Coconut scrapped 1 tbsp.
- Salt to taste

Method of preparation

- Soak the both brown and white rice overnight.
- Put the soaked rice in mixer or blender and add coconut, grind into smooth paste.
- Add required amount of salt.

- Heat the pan and smear little oil, take a ladle and mix it well. Take ladle full of batter and pour it over pan and spread it using back of ladle into round shape.
- Cover it for 1 min, add little oil and roast it according to your choice.
- Ready to eat Brown rice pancake

Benefits

- Brown rice is more nutritive rich in carbohydrates.
- When added with coconut it can build up tissues of body, impart strength, corrects bowel movements.
- Reduces *Vata dosha* thus builds up muscles and body strength.

GHEE ROAST PANCAKE

Ingredients

- White rice 1 cup
- Black gram split 2 tbsp.
- Fenugreek seeds ¼ tsp.
- Salt to taste

Method of preparation

1. Soak Rice, Black gram and fenugreek seeds for 4–5 hours in water.
2. Blend it In mixer to smooth paste adding little water, consistency needs to be thick.
3. Add little salt and stir it and keep it overnight to ferment.

4. Heat the pan smear little ghee, take a ladle and mix it well. Take ladle full of batter and pour it over pan and spread it using back of ladle into round shape.

5. Cover it for 1 min, add little ghee and roast it according to your choice.

Ready to eat ghee roast pancake.

Benefits

- Main ingredients of this ghee roast pan cake are rice and black gram.
- The ghee is added while roasting the pancake, which adds on to taste and health.
- Qualities of this food are, it is nourishing, neither light nor heavy so it is moderately digestive.
- This imparts nourishment, good built, strength to the body.
- It can be fed to babies by dipping it in milk or honey

Refer Fig 4.8

ONION PANCAKE

Ingredients

- Black gram 125 gms
- White rice 250 gms
- Onion 3 big
- Green chilly 2
- Ginger 1 inch
- Curry leaves 3 strands
- Salt to taste

Method of preparation

1. Soak black gram and rice for 2 hours.
2. Put this into mixer and grind it very finely.
3. The batter is kept overnight (next day it raises to double).
4. Next day morning add salt and mix thoroughly.
5. Finely chop onion, green chili, ginger.
6. Heat the pan and grease with little oil and spread the batter in circular form.
7. Add the chopped mixture on the batter and once the side is roasted flip the other side.

Benefits

- The ingredient of this being white rice, black gram and onion with carrot-ginger-chilly can be added as optional.
- As the mode of preparation is by roasting it on pan, it partly loses its heaviness and becomes moderately heavy which can be digested a easily.
- But it fills stomach soon as black gram is ingredient and pancake is thick.
- It increases strength, reduces *Vata dosha*, brings about better nutrition in thin person, it increases semen count in men.

Should be avoided

- In conditions such as skin disease, Obesity, poor digestive capacity, hyperacidity, Constipation.

Refer Fig 4.9

CUCUMBER PANCAKE (SWEET AND SPICY)

Ingredients for sweet pancake

- Rice 250 gms
- Coconut grated 2 fists
- Cucumber grated 1 medium
- Jaggery 1 cup (according to the level of sweet desired)

Method of preparation

1. Soak rice (white) for 2–3 hours.
2. Meanwhile squeeze the grated cucumber and remove excess water.
3. Grind the soaked rice along with grated coconut, make fine paste using the excess water from cucumber.
4. Add the grated jaggery and grated cucumber, mix well.
5. Heat the pan and spread the batter and flip over till properly cooked.

Benefits

- As cucumber is cool and light, this recipe can be often prepared in summer for people with excess body heat.
- Especially this pancake can be used in people with prickly heats, skin eruptions, people who often work in heated up atmosphere like road workers, building workers, fishermen as cools body very effectively

Refer Fig 5.0

SPICY CUCUMBER PANCAKE

Ingredients
- Rice 250 gms
- Coconut grated 2 fists
- Cucumber grated 1 medium
- Green chilies 1 (finely chopped)
- Pepper corn 2–3 (crushed)
- Cumin 1 tsp.

Method of preparation
1. Soak rice (white) for 2–3 hours.
2. Meanwhile squeeze the grated cucumber and remove excess water.
3. Grind the soaked rice along with grated coconut, make fine paste using the excess water from cucumber.
4. Add grated cucumber, finely chopped green chilies, pepper corn and cumin mix well.
5. Heat the pan and spread the batter and flip over till properly cooked.

Benefits
- Spicy cucumber pancake is more digestive.
- This can be used by people who don't prefer sweet, but this is less cooling that the sweet pancake.

SPICY PANCAKE

Ingredients
- Toor dal ½ cup
- White rice 1cup

- Red dry chilly 8
- Grated coconut ¼ cups
- Onion 2 big
- Cabbage 1 fist
- Tamarind little
- Oil
- Salt to taste

Method of preparation

1. Soak rice and toor dal for 2 hours, later wash it off.
2. Grind chili, tamarind and coconut with above soaked Ingredient. Make it a thick batter by adding medium water.
3. Transfer it into a bowl and add chopped onion and cabbage, salt and mix it well.
4. Heat the pan, add 2 spoon of oil and take batter and spread with bare hands over the heated pan.
5. In 1–2 min, sprinkle little oil over the pancake and flip it other side, both side should be cooked and roasted.

Variety

- Amaranth spicy pancake
- Same steps as simple spicy pancake replace onion and cabbage with amaranth leaves.

Benefits

- As it has good taste, it can be eaten in lunch time.
- People who have aversion towards sweets can eat this.
- People with high blood sugar level can eat this instead of sweet pancakes.

RICE DISHES

- GHEE RICE   317
- JEERA RICE   318
- MIXED VEGETABLE RICE   319
- MINT RICE   321
- TOMATO RICE   322
- CARROT RICE   323
- DIABETIC RICE   324

RICE DISHES

GHEE RICE

Ingredients

- Spices like bay leaf 1 in no., clove 3–4, and cardamom 2–3
- Ghee 2 tablespoon
- Onion/shallots: 1 big/4–5
- White rice (raw): 250 gms
- Pepper: optional

Method of preparation

1. Take a deep vessel and add ghee, once the ghee heats up add the spices in small quantities.
2. Add onion and roast till it turns golden color.
3. Add pepper and roast for a minute.
4. Now add rice and roast for about 3–4 minutes.
5. Add 500 ml of water or till the rice is completely dipped in water and add salt for taste.
6. Cook Profusely.

Garnish with coriander leaves or curry leaves.

Benefits

- Ghee rice is suitable in almost all types of body.
- It can be included in meal especially at lunch time.

- It is kind of cooling to the body as ghee is the main ingredient.
- It can be given to children and aged in little quantity.
- It is nourishing, easily digestible and enhances body strength.
- As in this spices are added in little quantity, the heaviness of rice and ghee is minimized.
- Hence it becomes easy to digest.

It should be avoided in the following conditions

- It should be avoided in conditions such as indigestion, Obesity, Diabetes.
- Person with lethargy, laziness, Irritable bowel syndrome should avoid eating this as after digestion, as it may worsen the above conditions.

JEERA RICE

Ingredients

- Oil/ghee: 2 table spoon
- Cumin (*Jeera*): 2 spoons
- Shallots: 3–5
- Rice (raw): 250 gms

Method of preparation

1. Take a deep vessel, add oil/ghee, and wait till it heats up.
2. Add shallots and roast it for 2 min.
3. Add cumin and roast till slight color change (2–3 min) in medium flame.
4. Now add the rice and roast it for 3–4 mins.

5. Add 500 ml of water or till the rice is completely dipped in water and add salt for taste.
6. Cook profusely.

Garnish it with curry leaves.

Benefits

- Cumin is one of the main ingredients and is good for digestion.
- It removes excess bloating of abdomen, cramps in muscles, eases the gastric disturbances in stomach
- It is light for digestion and easily absorbed by the body.
- It can be taken in medium quantity, even by children and the aged.

Refer Fig 5.1

MIXED VEGETABLE RICE

Ingredients

- Oil/ghee: 2 table spoon
- Spices like bay leaf (qty–1), cinnamon ½ inch stick, clove 1–2, cardamom 1–2
- Onion 1 big
- Vegetables like carrot, long green beans, green peas, cauliflower all together 200 gms
- Ginger garlic paste or pieces 1 tsp.
- Coriander leaves paste 2 tablespoon
- Turmeric powder ¼ tsp.

- All spices powder: ¼ tsp.
- Salt for taste

Method of preparation

1. Add oil/ghee in a deep pan, add spices and roast it for 30 sec.
2. Add onion and roast it for 2 min.
3. Add vegetables and roast it for 3–4 min.
4. Add turmeric and roast for 30 sec.
   - Add coriander paste and ginger-garlic paste to it, roast for 3–4 min.
5. Now add the rice and roast it for 3–4 min.
6. Add 500 ml of water or till the rice is completely dipped in water.
   - Add salt for taste.
7. Cook profusely.

Garnish with coriander leaves.

Benefits

- The dish mainly contains vegetables, so it is rich in fiber, vitamins and minerals.
- The ingredients such as oil/ghee, rice is heavy for digestion.
- But the ingredients such as ginger, garlic and spices makes it easy for digestion.
- It is better to avoid in individuals having Constipation, Acidity as the spices may cause sour belching and chest burn.

Refer Fig 5.

MINT RICE

Ingredients
- Oil/ghee: 1 tablespoon
- Mint leaves: 1 fist full
- Coriander leaves: ½ fist
- Spices like clove 1–2, pepper powder ¼ tsp.
- Onion 1 big
- Salt for taste

Method of preparation
1. Add oil/ghee in a deep pan, add spices and roast it for 30 sec.
2. Add onion and roast it for 2 min
3. Add paste of mint leaves, coriander and roast it for 3–4 min.
4. Now add rice and roast it for 3–4 min.
5. Add 500 ml of water or till the rice is completely dipped in water and add salt for taste.
6. Cook profusely.

Benefits
- Mint is the prime ingredient; hence it can be consumed in people with poor appetite, impaired digestion, and poor taste perception.
- It is good for joint problems, headaches, excessive body heat, hyperacidity (avoid adding spices, use shallots instead of onion).
- It should be taken with caution in people suffering from hyperacidity, Irritable bowel syndrome.
- Since the mint irritates the mucosa of alimentary tract.

Refer Fig 5.3

TOMATO RICE

Ingredients

- Oil/ghee: 1 tablespoon
- Spices like cinnamon ½ inch, garlic 2–3, ginger ½ inch
- Shallot: 5–6
- Turmeric: ¼ tsp.
- Pepper powder: ¼ tsp.
- Tomato: 2 big
- Salt for taste

Method of preparation

1. Add oil/ghee in a deep pan, add spices and roast it for 30 sec.
2. Add shallot and roast it for 2 min
3. Add turmeric and pepper powder
4. Add ginger and garlic roast for 1 min
5. Add tomato and cook for 3–4 min
6. Add white rice (raw) and roast for 2–3 min
7. Add 500 ml of water or till the rice is completely dipped in water.
    - Add salt for taste.
8. Cook it profusely.

Benefits

- In this recipe tomato is main ingredient, along with spices.
- Thus it is an appetizer, carminative and digestive.
- Tomato is good for enhancing vision, blood circulation,
- It should be avoided in people with Acidity, Urinary stones, Gall stone, Gouty arthritis, Psoriasis and Hyper sensitivity of skin or skin rashes.

CARROT RICE

Ingredients
- Oil/ghee: 1 tablespoon
- Spices bay leaf (qty–1) pepper powder 1/4 tsp., cumin seeds 7–8 no., cinnamon 1 inch stick
- Turmeric ¼ tsp.
- Onion 1 big
- Ginger garlic cut into small pieces 1 tsp.
- White rice (raw)
- Salt for taste

Method of preparation
1. Add oil/ghee in a deep pan, add spices and roast it for 30 sec.
2. Add shallot and roast it for 2 min.
3. Add turmeric and pepper powder.
4. Add ginger and garlic and roast it for 1 min.
5. Add carrot pieces and roast for 2–3 min.
    - Cook it for 3–4 min.
6. Add white rice (raw) and roast for 2–3 min.
7. Add 500 ml of water or till the rice is completely dipped in water and add salt for taste.
8. Cook it profusely.

Benefits
- In carrot rice, carrot is main ingredient along with ginger garlic and other spices, thus it is very good for digestion, and easily absorbed in the body.

- It should be avoided in Acidity, pain abdomen, and Irritable bowel as the carrot and spices mix would aggravate the condition by irritating mucosa of alimentary tract or by increasing the gastric secretion. Thus causes discomfort while and after digestion.

DIABETIC RICE

Ingredients

Note: Rice (Brown) which is stored for one year.
- i.e. 1 year old rice should be used.
- Rice: 200 gm. (old rice more than one year).
- Fenugreek: 5–6 should be taken.
- Water: 500 ml

Method of preparation
- The rice should be roasted lightly in a pan until it gets slightly brown.
- Then add water and fenugreek seeds, boil until properly cooked.

Benefits
- The rice helps to maintain blood sugar levels as well as give strength to body

DESSERTS

- CARROT HALWA — 327
- BANANA PUDDING — 328
- GUAVA HALWA — 328
- BEETROOT HALWA — 329
- ASH GOURD HALWA — 330
- PAPAYA HALWA — 331
- MANGO DELIGHT (AMRAS) — 332
- SEMOLINA PUDDING — 332

DESSERTS

CARROT HALWA

Ingredients
- Carrot 250 gms
- Milk 1cup
- Jaggery or sugar candy 3/4th cup
- Cardamom powder ½ tsp.
- Ghee ½ cup

Method of preparation

1. Clean the carrots and grate it.
   - Cook it with milk for 7–10 min or till it is cooked.
2. Add jaggery and stir it continuously, till the water content evaporates.
3. Add ghee and stir, later switch of the flame.
   - Sprinkle cardamom powder on it.

Benefits
- Carrot halwa contains all the ingredients that nourish the body.
- Carrot halwa cools down the increased body heat.
- It improves appetite, digestion, eye sight, and enhances skin texture.

Refer Fig 5.4

BANANA PUDDING

Ingredients
- Banana (qty - 4 big sizes)
- Jaggery 1cup
- Ghee 6 spoon
- Raisins 10
- Cashew nuts 10
- Cardamom powder 1/2 tsp.

Method of preparation
1. Peel off the skin of banana and cut it into small pieces.
2. Take a deep bottom vessel and add ghee, also add banana pieces and stir it for 5 min.
3. Add jaggery and keep stirring till it leaves the sides of the pan.
4. Add roasted raisins and cashew nuts and stir again and sprinkle cardamom powder.

Benefits
- Banana is rich in vitamin, minerals and thus has multiple effect.
- When added with other sweetening agents, ghee becomes very much nutritious and builds the body.
- Good in acidity problems, weakness or debility, improves digestion.

GUAVA HALWA

Ingredients
- Guava 3 medium sized
- Sugar candy

- Water
- Cardamom 1/2 tsp.
- Lemon 1

Method of preparation

1. Cut the extras of guava, wash it and cook with water (the guava must be covered with water) for 7–8 min.
2. Remove the cooked guava and grind it into paste and sieve it.
3. Add sugar candy equal to the quantity of guava paste and cook with continuous stirring till it bubbles (7–10 min).
4. Switch off the flame and then add lemon juice and cardamom powder.
5. Grease a plate with ghee and pour the above paste into it.
6. After 4–5 hours, it solidifies, and then can be cut into pieces with knife.

Benefits

- Guava is best supplement for Vitamin C, has good impact on improving vision, even does normalize thyroid hormone.
- It improves brain growth and helpful in cancer
- It can be eaten by person with *Vata* and *Pitha* dosha.

BEETROOT HALWA

Same method as carrot halwa but replaces carrot with beetroots.

Benefits

- Beetroot is best in Constipation, for skin health, blood purifier, and aphrodisiac.

- It is also good in blood pressure management and in brain function enhancement.
- It can be eaten with person of all three *Vata, Pitha,* and *Kapha doshas.*

ASH GOURD HALWA

Ingredients

- Ash gourd 1 medium size
- Saffron strands 3–4
- Ghee 6 spoons
- Jaggery ¾ of the quantity of ash gourd
- Cardamom 1/4 tsp.

Method of preparation

1. Grate the ash gourd and cook it
2. As the water start evaporating add jaggery, keep stirring, as it gets dried or much of evaporated add 2 spoon ghee.
3. Sprinkle cardamom and saffron and stir continuously, then add remaining 2 spoon of ghee and stir.

Benefits

- Ash gourd is a best in building body mass, in respiratory diseases, bleeding disorders.
- It builds up a strong immune system.

PAPAYA HALWA

Ingredients

- Papaya 1 big
- Milk 2 cup
- Jaggery 2 cups
- Ghee ½ cup
- Cardamom ¼ tsp.

Method of preparation

1. Yellow colored papaya medium riped, peel off the skin and remove seeds, cut into small pieces.
2. Cook it with milk, till the papaya gets soft.
3. The papaya should grind properly.
4. Add jaggery to above mixture and stir it continuously on medium flame.
5. After it leaves the sides of pan, add ghee and stir continuously.
6. Transfer it to a plate greased with ghee and check if it is sticky, if it is not sticky then the halwa preparation is right, if sticky cook further till stickiness disappears.
7. Add cardamom and stir.

Benefits

- Papaya is best for skin and digestive tract, it helps relieve Constipation.
- It is best in degenerative diseases, as it prevents further degeneration.
- It is good in irregular menstrual problems.
- It builds up a stronger immune system.

MANGO DELIGHT (AMRAS)

Ingredients

- Ripened mango 2
- Coconut milk 250 ml
- Sugar 6–7 spoons
- Cardamom ¼ tsp.

Method of preparation

1. Extract the juice from the ripened mango, by squeezing.
2. Add coconut milk to mango juice.
3. Add sugar and mix thoroughly.
4. Sprinkle cardamom powder.

Benefits

- Same as mango juice.

SEMOLINA PUDDING

Ingredients

- Semolina 1 cup
- Milk
- Water
- Jaggery
- Ghee
- Cardamom
- Raisins/cashew
- Saffron

Method of preparation

1. Roast semolina in a pan, till it starts emitting roasted smell.
   - Please do not roast it till brown.
   - Transfer it to a separate container.
2. In same pan add ghee (1 tbsp.) fry cashews and raisins. Set them aside.
3. Add water in the pan with few saffron strands and boil it.
   - Add roasted semolina to it, cook it and keep stirring.
   - Add milk to it.
4. Once semolina is cooked, add jaggery and ghee and keep stirring.
5. Turn off the gas and garnish with roasted cashews and raisins.

Benefits

- It provides energy to body and can be given to babies, as it is easy to digest.
- It is a good antioxidant, and good for muscle cramps.
- It has good content of calcium in it, thus makes the bone stronger.

Refer Fig 5.5

SWEET PUDDINGS

- RICE PUDDING — 337
- VERMICELLI PUDDING — 338
- BROKEN WHEAT PUDDING — 338
- RAVA PUDDING — 339
- BENGAL GRAM PUDDING — 340
- JACKFRUIT PUDDING/JACKFRUIT DESSERT — 340
- SWEET PONGAL — 341
- BENEFITS OF ALL SWEET PUDDINGS — 343

SWEET PUDDINGS

RICE PUDDING

Ingredients

- White Rice (raw) 150 gm
- Jaggery 150 gms
- Grated coconut 1 cup
- Cardamom ¼ tsp.
- Raisins 6–7

Method of preparation

1. Wash and drain the white raw rice and boil it with enough water.
2. When the rice is boiling, take grated coconut and grind it until the milk comes out of it.
   - Keep the thick milk and thin milk separately.
3. As the water is evaporating from the boiling rice, add thin coconut milk and boil further.
4. Once the rice is boiled add jaggery to it and cover it with lid.
5. After two boils add thick coconut milk.
   - Once it again boils, switch off the flame.
   - Later add cardamom powder and raisins.

VERMICELLI PUDDING

Ingredients
- Vermicelli 150 gms
- Coconut milk 500 ml
- Sugar 150 gms
- Ghee 100 gms
- Cardamom powder 1/4 tsp.
- Cashew and raisins 6–7 each

Method of preparation
1. Take ghee in a pan, heat it. Roast the vermicelli till it emits smell.
2. Add water and cook, till its soft.
3. Add sugar and stir it.
4. Add coconut milk and boil it for 5–6 min.
5. If it is very thick, add a little water and make it porridge consistency.

Refer Fig 5.6

BROKEN WHEAT PUDDING

Ingredients
- Broken wheat 150 gms
- Jaggery 300 gms
- Coconut milk of 1 medium sized coconut
- Cashew
- Cardamom ¼ tsp.
- Salt 1 pinch

Method of preparation

1. Cook broken wheat with enough water.
2. To this, add jaggery and a pinch of salt.
3. Once the jaggery melts and a boil appears.
    - Add coconut milk to it.
4. Boil it till 5–8 min.
    - Broken wheat pudding is ready to serve.

RAVA PUDDING

Ingredients

- Semolina
- Ghee
- Sugar
- Coconut milk
- Cardamom
- Cashew

Method of preparation

1. Heat the ghee in deep bottom pan.
    - Roast semolina till it turns golden brown color.
2. Add coconut milk and cook it completely.
3. Add sugar and cook for 2–3 min.
4. Sprinkle cardamom powder.
    - Rava pudding is ready to serve.

BENGAL GRAM PUDDING

Ingredients

- Split Bengal gram 50 g
- Coconut milk 150 ml
- Jaggery 90 gm
- Cardamom 1/4 tsp.
- Ghee 1 tbsp.
- Raisins 7–8
- Cashew 5–6

Method of preparation

1. Soak Bengal gram for 1/hour.
2. Cook Bengal gram in 120 ml of water till it becomes soft.
3. Add jaggery and mix until it melts.
4. Add coconut milk to above mixture and keep boiling until it turns thick.
5. Cashew and raisins should be slightly roasted in ghee and added to the above mixture.
6. Sprinkle cardamom.
    - Bengal gram pudding is ready to serve.

JACKFRUIT PUDDING/JACKFRUIT DESSERT

Ingredients

- Ripe jackfruit 10 pieces
- Jaggery ½ cup
- Water ¼ cup
- Coconut milk ¾ cup

- Cashew nuts 4–5
- Coconut bits 1 tbsp.
- Cardamom powder pinch

Method of preparation

1. Cook jackfruit in pressure cooker with water level just so that the jackfruit immerse a bit.
   - Cook for 2 whistles and allow to cool and drain it. Grind it into fine paste in a mixer.
2. Mix jaggery with ¼ cup of water, stir it and strain to remove impurities. Heat it until it bubbles.
3. To the above mixture add grinded jackfruit paste and mix evenly until it mixes up.
4. As it becomes thick, add ghee and mix it. Later mix the coconut milk in it and stir.
   - Don't allow it to boil. So when the mixture is about to boil, switch it off.
   - Roast cashew and coconut bits in ghee till it turns slight brown.
   - Add cardamom for garnishing.
   - Jackfruit dessert is ready to eat.

SWEET PONGAL

Ingredients

- White rice ½ cup
- Green gram (split) ½ cup
- Grated jaggery ½ cup
- Cardamom powder 1 pinch

- Ghee 2–3 tablespoon
- Raisins 5–6
- Cashew 7–8
- Clove 1–2
- Coconut pieces chopped: few

Method of preparation

1. Roast green gram in a pan until it emits fragrance, add rice to the same pan.
2. Wash them twice.
3. Then pour 2 cups of water, now cook these together in a pressure cooker for 2 whistles.
4. Take jaggery, add ¼ cup of water to it. Stir it over low flame and melt it.
5. Mash the cooked mixture of rice and green gram slightly.
6. Filter the jaggery syrup and add it to the cooked mixture.
7. Sprinkle cardamom powder, mix well and cook on medium flame till jaggery mixes up well.
8. Then the above mixture will begin to bubble well. Then turn it off.
9. In other pan, heat ghee. Add coconut pieces, fry till they turn aromatic.
10. Then add it to the rice mixture.
11. Roast cashew, clove and add raisins. Mix this with rice.

Sweet pongal is ready to eat.

Refer Fig 5.7

BENEFITS OF ALL SWEET PUDDINGS

- Sweet puddings are generally nourishing, highly nutritious as ingredients such as milk, jaggery, and dry fruits are used in it.
- It is pleasing to taste buds and mind.
- It promotes weight gain.
- It builds up the body tissues, good for heart, Hypertension.
- Basically all the sweet puddings are good in persons with *Pitha* and *Vata doshas*.

SWEET DRINKS

- BANANA MILK DRINK　　　　　　　　　　　　347
- MANGO DRINK　　　　　　　　　　　　　　347
- MUSK MELON DRINK　　　　　　　　　　　348

SWEET DRINKS

BANANA MILK DRINK

Ingredients
- Banana 4–5 medium sized
- Coconut milk
- Sugar

Method of preparation
1. Cut banana into small pieces and then mash few.
2. Grind the mashed ones with the coconut milk.
3. Add few pieces of banana into the grinded mixture.
4. Add cashew, cardamom, sugar in the end.

Benefits
- Banana is the best supplement for calcium, potassium and coconut milk is best for skin and hairs.
- This combination is best nourishing drink, best in people with thin body and dry skin.

MANGO DRINK

Ingredients
- Ripened mango 4–5 medium sized
- Coconut milk
- Sugar

Method of preparation

1. Cut Mango into small pieces and then mash few.
2. Grind the mashed ones with the coconut milk.
3. Add few pieces of Mango into the grinded mixture.
4. Add cashew, cardamom, sugar in the end.

Benefits

- The drink is a good antioxidant.
- It contains sour and sweet taste; hence it is best in heart related disorders.
- It improves digestion and is good for vision.
- It promotes brain health, regulates blood pressure, enhance skin health, improves immunity.

MUSK MELON DRINK

Ingredients

- Musk melon 4–5 medium sized
- Coconut milk
- Sugar

Method of preparation

1. Cut Musk melon into small pieces and then mash a few.
2. Grind the mashed ones with the coconut milk.
3. Add few pieces of Musk melon and sugar into the grinded mixture.

Benefits

- The drink is the best supplement for Vitamin and potassium.
- Hence it is best in vision problems, Hypertension or increased blood pressure.
- As the fruit is free from cholesterol it can be consumed by people with high cholesterol.
- It is the best coolant and helps in soothing stomach ulcer, relieves constipation, also brings down menstrual cramps.
- It is best for skin, hairs, heart.

NON VEGETARIAN DISHES

CHICKEN RECIPES

- CHICKEN APPETIZER SOUP — 353
- STRENGTHENING SOUP (MUTTON) — 354
- CHICKEN COCONUT DELIGHT — 355
- CHICKEN CURRY — 357

FISH RECIPES

- FISH CLAY POT CURRY — 359
- FISH COCONUT DELIGHT — 361
- FISH PAN FRY — 362

NON VEGETARIAN DISHES

CHICKEN APPETIZER SOUP

Ingredients

- Chicken 1 boneless chicken breast
- Onion 1 (to be cut into medium pieces)
- Ginger 1 inch (to be cut into small pieces)
- Carrot 1 (to be cut into medium pieces)
- Water ½ liter
- Pepper as per personal taste
- Salt for taste
- Coriander leaves for garnish

Method of preparation

1. Pour water in deep bottom vessel and cook vegetables along with ginger.
2. In the other pan, cook chicken about 10 min or until it is properly cooked
3. Once the chicken is cooked, chop it into small pieces,
   - On the other hand when the vegetables are cooked, drain them.
4. The stock (water in which vegetables are cooked) is to be taken in a pan.
   - Add the chicken pieces, salt as per taste and boil it on low flame.
5. Garnish it with coriander leaves.

Benefits

- It is useful as an appetizer in person who has less hunger, who is thin or lost weight.
- This soup can be taken with more pepper and spices, if a person has cold.
- Chicken soup is beneficial in person with *Vata dosha* predominance, and in muscle weakness, fatigue syndrome.

STRENGTHENING SOUP (MUTTON)

Ingredients

- Mutton 200 gms
- Onion 1
- Tomato 1
- Garlic 6–7 clove
- Cumin 1 tbsp.
- A pinch of pepper corn
- Green chilli 2
- Coriander leaves to garnish
- Salt for taste

Method of preparation

1. Cut the onion into thick pieces and grind it along with garlic, pepper, cumin in the mixer.
   - Make it into paste.
2. Take cleaned mutton pieces preferably mutton leg.
   - Place it in pressure cooker along with paste, tomato, green chilies, and salt.

3. Cook it for until 2–3 whistles.
4. When cooked remove the lid.
   - Add some oil (3 tsp.) and boil for few minutes.
5. Finally garnish with coriander leaves, one can add extra pepper if one desires.

Benefits

- Strengthening mutton soup is best for good nourishment hence given in thin and weak people.
- It should be taken by person with good digestive power or they have chances of having indigestion.
- It is best supplement of calcium and iron thus can be taken in Osteoarthritis, fracture, anemia, increases the blood count.
- This soup is best for males to increase sexual capacity.

Refer Fig 5.8

CHICKEN COCONUT DELIGHT

Ingredients

- For roasting
- Coriander seeds 1½ tsp.
- Cumin seeds ½ tsp.
- Fenugreek seeds ¼ tsp.
- Cinnamon 1 inch
- Clove 4–5
- Fennel seeds ¼ tsp.
- Pepper corn 5–6

- Turmeric powder ¼ tsp.
- Roast all these ingredients
- Dry red chilies 5–6 (To be Roasted separately)
- Chicken 500 gms
- Onion 2 (big in size)
- Garlic 5–6 clove
- Grated coconut ½ cups
- Curry leaves 1 sprig
- Tamarind 1 lemon sized
- Tomato 1 medium
- Oil/Ghee 2–3 tbsp.
- Salt for taste
- Paste of garlic and onion (1) is to be made in the mixer.
- Later add coconut and run the mixer for 4–5 sec (so that coconut doesn't turn into fine paste)

Method of preparation

1. The ingredients mentioned under roasting should be roasted till brown.
    - All the spices roasted first and red chilies roasted separately till it becomes crisp (light brown).
2. Once the above roasted ingredients cool, powder until it becomes fine powder in a mixer.
3. In a deep bottom pan, heat the oil with few curry leaves, onion (long sliced).
    - Fry till it becomes slight golden color.
    - Add sliced tomato, cleaned chicken (medium sized pieces) and cook for 5 min with lid closed.

4. Now add the roasted powder and mix it properly.
   - Add little water about 150 ml.
   - Boil chicken for 15 min, with lid closed.
5. Once chicken is almost cooked, add the coconut paste and cook for 10 min with closed lid. (Add water if required, it shouldn't be dry while cooking)
6. Add the tamarind water, little salt and cook for 7 min on medium flame. (Stir on regular intervals)
7. Add remaining curry leaves and switch it off.

Benefits
- It is very tasty and healthy as it contains mixture of spices and coconut.
- It is nourishing and easy for digestion.
- It enhances body built and also good for sexual capacity.

Refer Fig 5.9

CHICKEN CURRY

Ingredients

Marinate
- Chicken 500 gms (cut into medium pieces)
- Red chili powder ¼ tsp.
- Turmeric ¼ tsp.
- Lemon juice 1 tbsp.(optional)
- Pepper powder ¼ tsp.
- All spices powder ¼ tsp.

Spices to roast

- Coriander seeds 1 ½ tbsp.
- Cumin seeds ¼ tsp.
- Fennel seeds 4–5
- Pepper powder ¼ tsp.
- Cinnamon tick 1 inch
- Clove 4
- Red chilies 2–3
- Roast it till crisp or slight brown and grind with enough water to make paste.

Gravy

- Onion sliced ½ cup
- Ginger garlic paste 1 tbsp.
- Coconut milk ¾ cup
- Coconut oil 1 ½ tbsp.
- Season with
- Coconut oil 1 tsp.
- 1 red chili
- Shallots 2–3
- Curry leaves 1 small piece

Method of preparation

1. Marinate chicken with above ingredients for 40–50 min.
2. Dry, roast the spices and makes it into powder.
    - And to the powder, add little water and make into smooth paste.

3. Heat coconut oil in a deep bottom pan, add onions. Fry it till it becomes golden.
4. Add the ginger garlic paste; fry till raw smell goes off.
5. Add chicken and roast for 3–4 min.
6. Pour the spice paste and mix well and cook over medium flame. Cook till the chicken is soft.
7. Add coconut milk and mix well. It begins to boil, bubble and simmer, cook for 5–6 min.
8. Heat coconut oil in pan add shallots, curry leaves and season the curry.

Benefits
- This curry is very healthy and easy to digest.
- It gives good nourishment and is easily absorbed in the body.
- It can also be taken with rice, chapathi and rice pan cake.

Refer Fig 6.0

FISH CLAY POT CURRY

Ingredients
- Fish 200 gms
- Dry red chili 4–5
- Garlic cloves 5
- Curry leaves 10
- Tamarind lemon sized pulp (soaked in 2 cups of hot water)
- Coriander powder 1 tbsp.

- Turmeric powder 1 tbsp.
- Fenugreek seeds 1 tsp.
- Pepper powder ½ tsp.
- Cumin powder ½ tsp.
- Green chilies 2
- Salt as per taste
- Onion 2 medium size
- Tomato 1 large finely chopped
- Coconut oil 1 tbsp.

Method of preparation

1. Grind red chilies and garlic into a fine paste.
2. Squeeze the tamarind well and obtain the thick juice.
3. Mix the red chili paste and tamarind juice with turmeric and coriander powder with salt.
4. Place pot on the stove, add oil and wait then increase flame to medium.
   - Add curry leaves and fenugreek seeds, green chilies, salt for 2 min.
5. Add the paste of onion and stir it, let it cook for 5–7 min.
6. Add chopped tomatoes and stir till it completely cooks.
7. Later add the extracted tamarind juice, cook with lid closed.
   - Cook till the curry starts boiling lightly.
8. Add pepper and cumin powder. Cook for about 5–7 min.
9. Add fish and cook till done.

Note

- Don't stir much after the fish is added, as stirring much would break it into pieces.

- Keep the lid closed for about 30 min after switching off the gas before serving.

Benefits

- This curry is rich in Omega 3 fatty acids and even minerals as it is made in clay pot.
- Fish curry doesn't increase the fat or cholesterol as it is rich in spices.
- Easy to digest and can be had in meal time with rice.

Refer Fig 6.1

FISH COCONUT DELIGHT

Ingredients

- Fish sardine 500 gms
- Shallots 250 gms
- Ginger 1 tbsp.
- Green chilies 3
- Tamarind 2 inch long
- Coconut 1 cup
- Turmeric powder ½ tsp.
- Coconut oil 1 tbsp.
- Salt to taste

Method of preparation

1. Clean the fish and cut it into small pieces.
2. Grated coconut, sliced onion, chopped ginger, crushed green chillis, turmeric powder should be mixed in a bowl and slightly pressed with hand.

3. In a clay pot or a normal deep bottom vessel put fish pieces with salt, tamarind and coconut mixture. Mix well.

4. Add little water and cook over medium flame with closed lid until the water is reduced or nearly evaporated about 7–10 min

5. Sprinkle 1 tbsp.of coconut oil just before switching off the flame.

Benefits

- This is good for digestion and a tasty delight.
- Coconut and tamarind being main ingredient, it nourishes body and provides smoothness to skin and hair.

Refer Fig 6.2

FISH PAN FRY

Ingredients

- Fish (sardine, mackerel, seer fish) 500 gms
- Red chili powder 2–3 tsp.
- Tamarind pulp marble sized
- Pepper powder ½ tsp.
- Garlic 2–3 clove
- Oil 3–4 tbsp.
- Salt to taste

Method of preparation

1. Grind all the ingredients together with very little water to make a thick paste.

2. Marinate the fishes with the chili paste above for about 40–60 min.

3. Heat the oil in a flat or medium shallow pan
4. Add the marinated fish and fry it on both sides about 4 min each side or till roasted.

Benefits

- Usually fish is baked or deep fried which is not good for health.
- Here the fish is roasted with less oil and it contains mixture of spices, so it is good for people with cholesterol.
- Can be made less spicy and consumed.

Refer Fig 6.3

AYURVEDA HOME REMEDIES

- COLD/COUGH/SORE THROAT/TONSILITTIS/FEVER — 367
- STOMACH ACHE — 368
- SKIN ITCHING — 368
- WEIGHT LOSS — 368
- HAIR LOSS — 369
- HEADACHE/MIGRAINE — 369
- ACNE/PIMPLES — 370
- CONSTIPATION — 370
- DIARRHOEA — 371

AYURVEDA HOME REMEDIES

COLD/COUGH/SORE THROAT/TONSILITTIS/FEVER

1. Long pepper powder is made into fine powder and kept ready. 2–3 grams of the powder is mixed with honey and licked. This relieves Cough, Cold, sore throat.
2. Powder of long pepper is made and soaked with hot water in the ratio of 1:4 and kept for a while. This is to be taken by mixing 1 spoon of ghee, in lukewarm condition twice daily. Effective for sore throat and Tonsillitis. Dose: 30–50 ml.
3. Basil leaves few in number with little bit turmeric should be boiled with ginger tea .Drink warm cup of this tea every 3–4 hours for fever, cold.
4. Ginger and honey should be taken in equal quantity, mixed well. Later boiled for few seconds. Take a teaspoon of this mixture and lick it thrice a day for cough and cold
5. Turmeric one tablespoon and black pepper should be mixed with into a glass of warm milk. Mix properly and drink it. Do it twice a day to get relief from cold and fever.

STOMACH ACHE

1. Take pomegranate seed applied with some black salt and pepper corn powder. It is very useful in stomach ache.
2. Take equal quantity of ginger and mint extract and mix little bit rock salt to give maximum relief in stomach ache as well as vomiting also.
3. Chew some roasted fennel seeds in stomach ache or abdominal pain.
    - Mix coriander powder with sugar candy to stop stomach ache or abdominal pain.
4. Prepare the powder of cumin seeds and daily use 2–3 times with warm water to get relief from stomach ache.

SKIN ITCHING

1. Mix lemon juice in jasmine oil and massage on itching skin.
2. Mix lemon juice in coconut oil and apply to stop itching.
3. Massage with peel of orange on the skin and get rid of skin itching.
4. Daily use 20 gram of honey with cool water.

WEIGHT LOSS

1. Normal water should be mixed with honey and taken in empty stomach.
2. Lemon juice should be taken with warm water in empty stomach.
3. Cinnamon powder is to be boiled in one cup of water and after cooling mix one spoon of honey. Drink in morning in breakfast, and before sleeping.

4. Salad of tomato and onion should be taken daily with meal. Mix salt and squeeze lemon extract for better results.

HAIR LOSS

1. Indian gooseberry 5–6 tablespoon should be mixed with 5–6 tablespoon of water.
   - Make it into paste and apply to scalp and hair. Leave it for 30 minutes and then wash off with shampoo.
   - Do this thrice a week.
2. Fenugreek seeds 2 tablespoon should be roasted in a pan and then grinded into fine powder. Add some water to make it into paste.
   - Apply on scalp and leave it for 20 minutes. Later wash off with shampoo.
   - Do this twice a week.
3. Aloe Vera gel half cup with 3 tablespoon of coconut oil and 2 tablespoon of honey should be combined to get a consistent mixture. Apply to this scalp and hair for 30 minutes. Later wash off with this shampoo.

HEADACHE/MIGRAINE

1. Dried ginger should be roasted with butter, tie in soft handkerchief or cotton cloth and sniff it to get quick relief from migraine headaches.
2. Fresh Basil leaves can be put in boiling water or tea and drink it when it is lukewarm.

3. Pepper mint oil can be massaged on forehead and neck. Or smell the oil for few minutes to get relief from headache.
4. Crushed ginger (small piece) and basil leaves should be added into a cup of boiling water, add some milk and sugar. Drink it after it becomes lukewarm.

ACNE/PIMPLES

1. Garlic cloves 2–3 should be crushed to make a paste. Apply to affected area. If skin is sensitive mix yoghurt in garlic paste before applying.
2. Take handful of washed coriander leaves, crush them finely. Place the paste of sieve and press to extract juice.
   - Add pinch of turmeric powder and mix well.
   - Apply on face every night.
3. Turmeric paste with warm water should be applied, once dried it can be rubbed off.
   - One can replace turmeric with honey for dry skin.
4. Lemon juice should be directly to the pimple overnight.
5. Wash face, pat dry and apply papaya paste on face. Leave the mask for 20–30 minutes.

CONSTIPATION

1. Soak dry grapes 10–15 over night and take empty stomach.
2. Dry fig also can be done in the same way.
3. Fenugreek seeds soaked in water overnight and taken in morning empty stomach.
4. Flax seeds with warm water should be taken in empty stomach.

DIARRHOEA

1. Pomegranate seeds boiled in water and filtered should be taken 2–3 times per day.
2. Banana should be taken with buttermilk.
3. Cumin seeds with honey.
4. Honey with cold water.
5. Mint leaf juice 5–6 times daily.

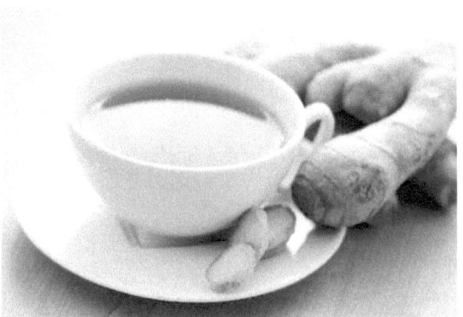

Fig 3.9 Ginger Water

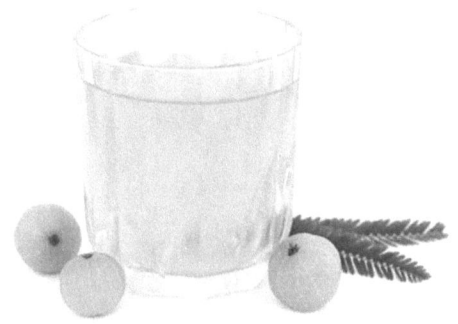

Fig 4.0 Amla Juice

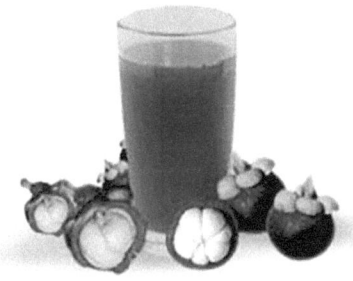

Fig 4.1 Cocum Juice

Fig 4.2 Tomato Soup

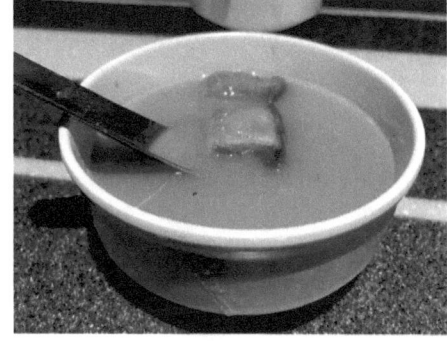

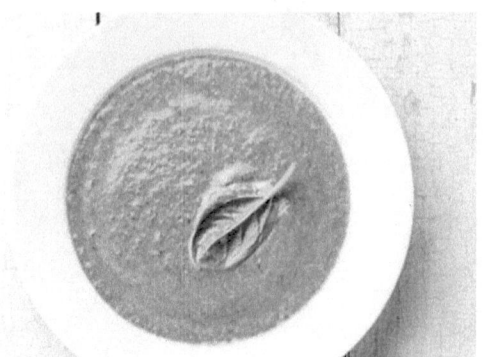

Fig 4.3 Spinach Soup

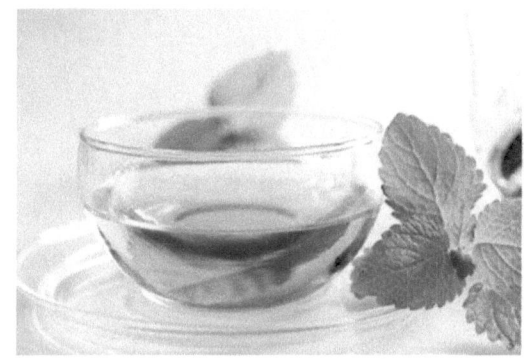

Fig 4.4 Tulasi Tea

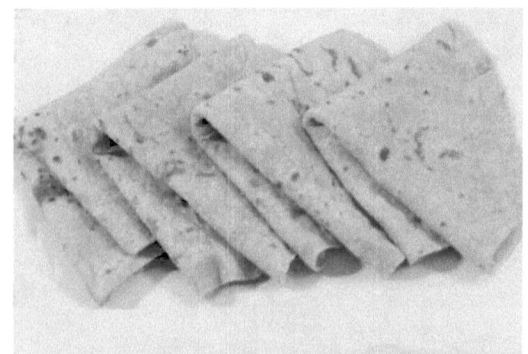

Fig 4.5 Chapathi

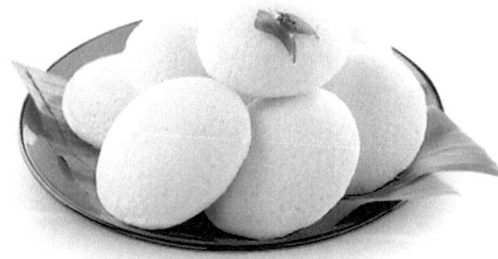

Fig 4.6 Idly

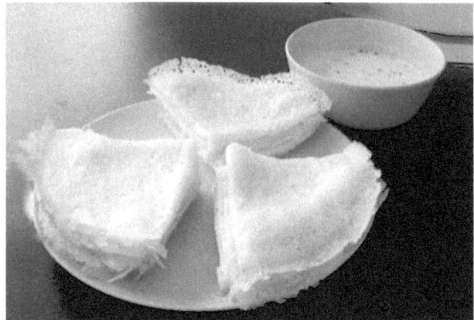

Fig 4.7 Rice Pancake

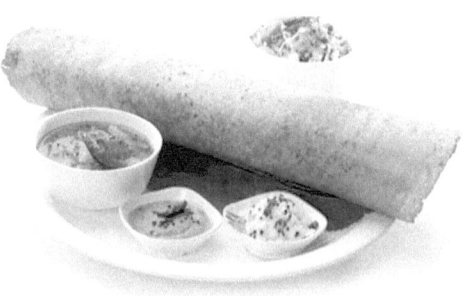

Fig 4.8 Ghee Roast Pan Cake

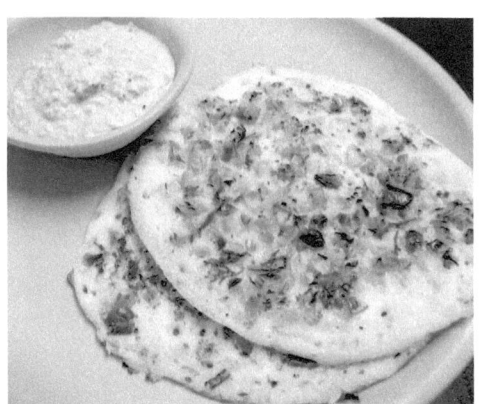

Fig 4.9 Onion Pancake

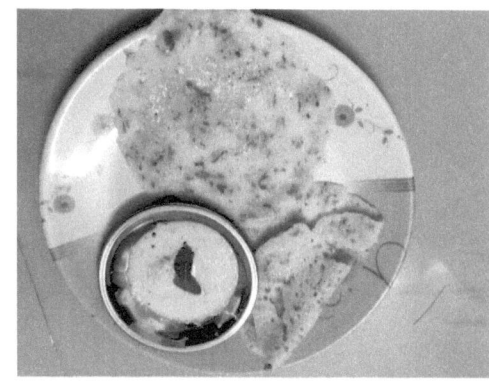

Fig 5.0 Cucumber Pancake

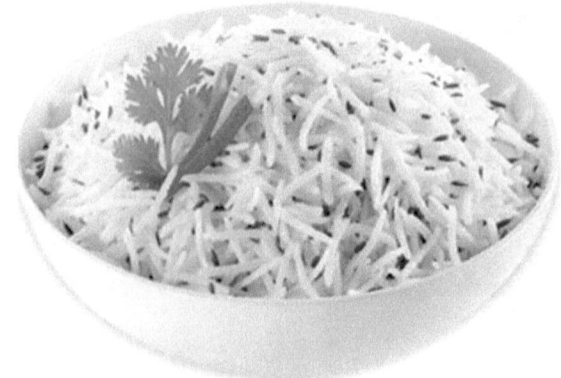

Fig 5.1 Jeera Rice

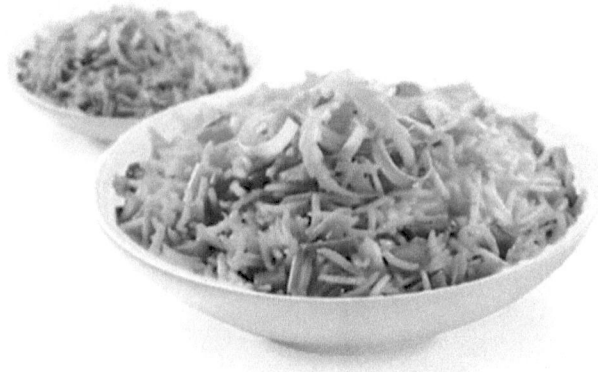

Fig 5.2 Mixed Vegetable Rice

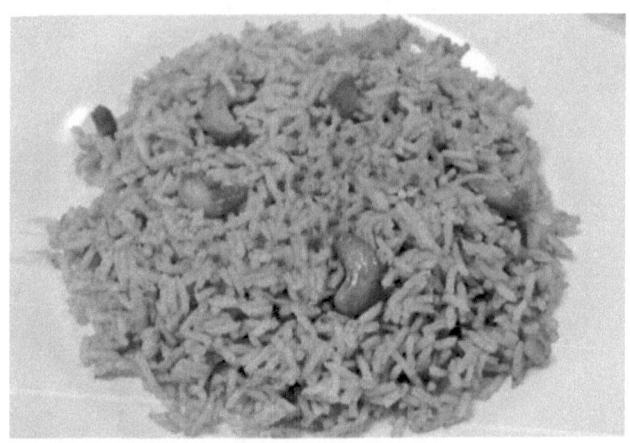

Fig 5.3 Mint Rice

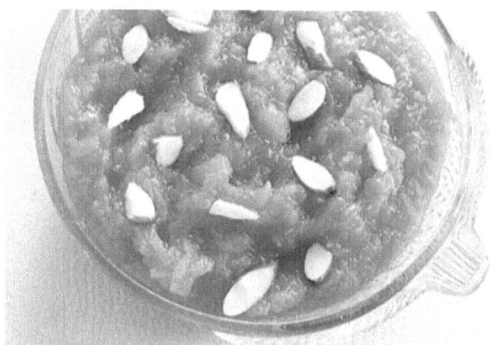

Fig 5.4 Carrot Halwa

Fig 5.5 Semolina Pudding

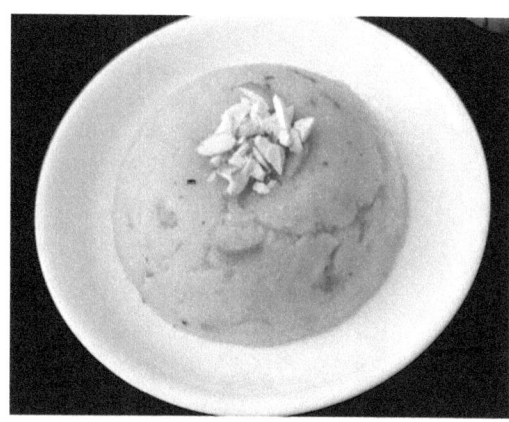

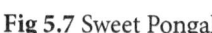

Fig 5.6 Vermicelli Pudding

Fig 5.7 Sweet Pongal

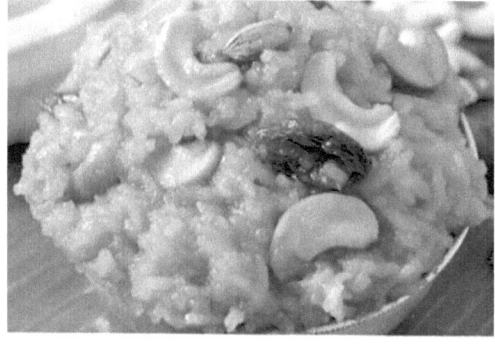

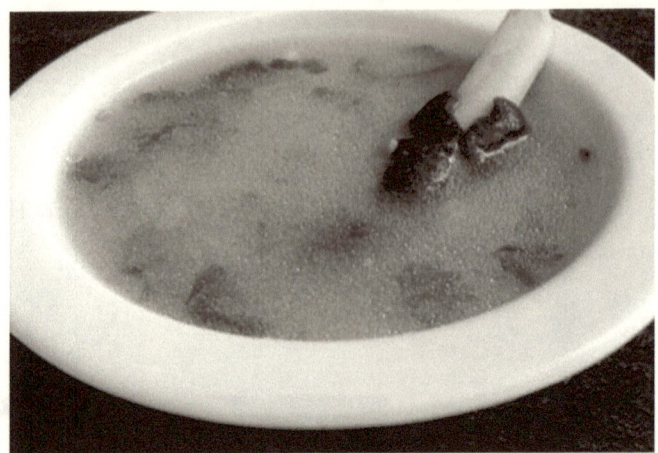

Fig 5.8 Strengthening Soup

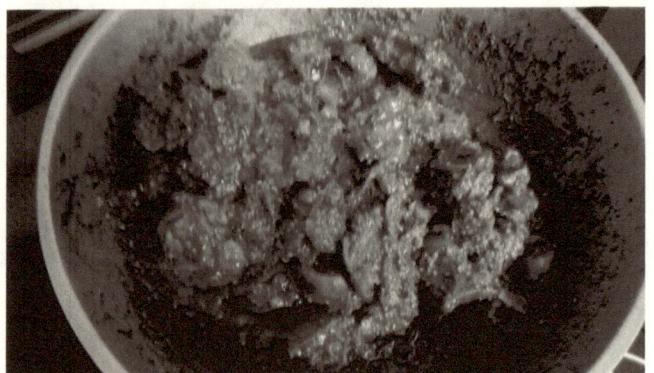

Fig 5.9 Chickeen Cocunut Delight

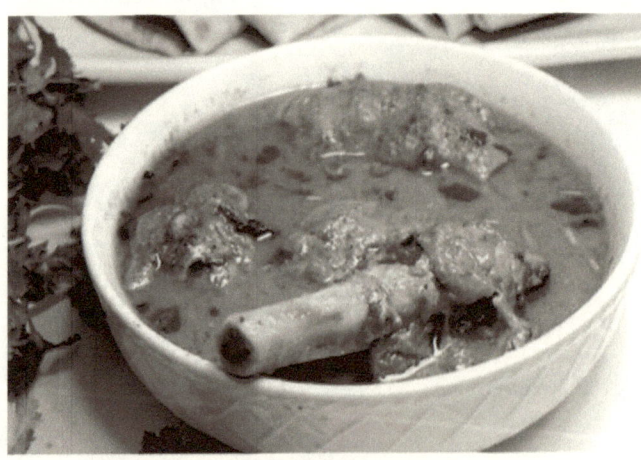

Fig 6.0 Chicken Curry

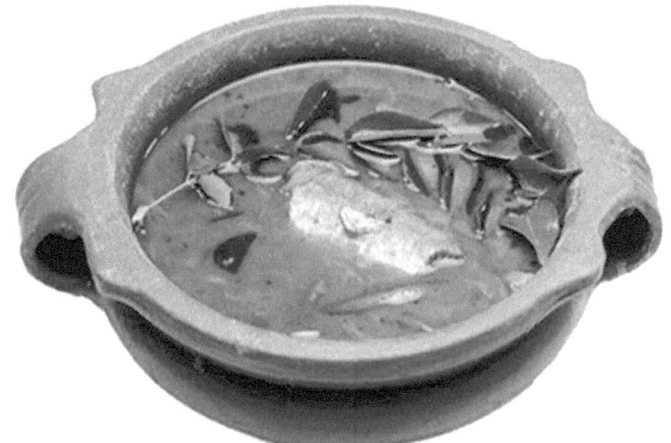

Fig 6.1 Fish Clay Pot Curry

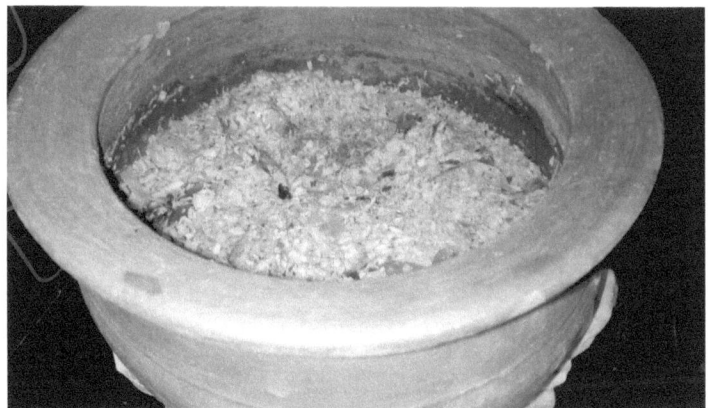

Fig 6.2 Fish Cocunut Delight

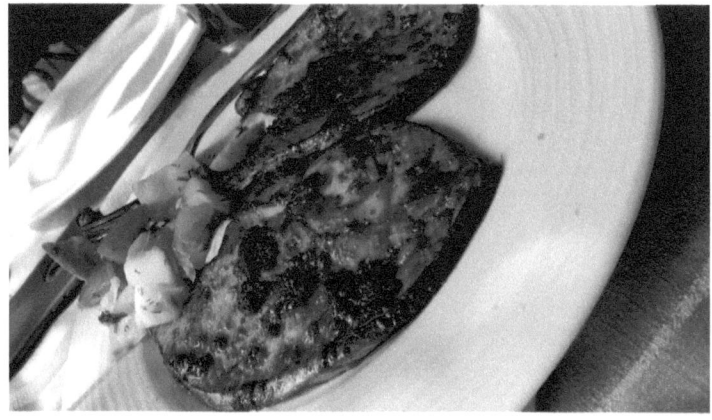

Fig 6.3 Fish Pan Fry

DEAR READERS

- In the book I have described Ayurveda in the simplest and practical way.
- Start applying Ayurveda in your life today, Tomorrow might never come.
- Throughout the book I have tried to convey the message about nurturing health by avoiding unhealthy practices in your life.
- Ayurveda is not only about curative or preventive factor for disease, but it teaches the way of living.
- By following Ayurveda one can live a healthy life, rather than depending on medicines.
- Stop harming yourself, your health and life.
- Wake up!! Realize and start today before it is too late!
- The herbs, medicines and any other food mentioned here are available in India.

ACHIEVEMENTS

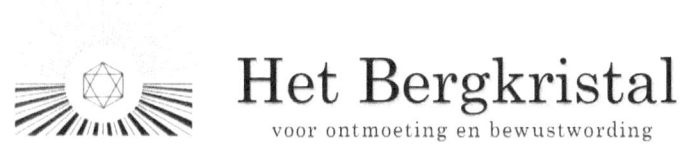

Het Bergkristal
voor ontmoeting en bewustwording

Belversestraat 40
5076 PZ Haaren
tel: 0411-621003
info@bergkristal.nl
www.bergkristal.nl
NL40TRIO0197886981
t.n.v. Stichting de Lightberg
KvK: 41055466

Haaren 15-08-2017

DcDr Raj Mohan in The Netherlands- Bergkristal Haaren (NB)
Worshops ayurvedic health care and way of living / consultations
9-14 juli 2017

Hello Dr RajMohan :

We enjoyed you're stay with us. You have an open en beautiful caracter> It was very nice that you were talking to all the people. You are a very inspired person wth wisdom.

You had your well prepared for the workshop and your openness was very good. You picked the good feedback on and you had well prepared with your PowerPoint presentation schedules, you transfer was clear.
The 30 persons who came to you'r workshops were very happy with you're information and presentations and that they became it afterwards in their mail box, for reading!

The people were excited with you're consultations with personal open attention and care.

A beautiful shape was the interaction with your audience, what you more did, where by the people are going to feel more a part of what you're talking about and sharing.

It was nice to see that you too are curious about us, our culture, customs, society and language. We are happy that we have been able to experience various aspects there of.

Give your goal and desire confidence, there is a way. With You're personality you will succeed to bring you're expertice abroad and to Europe !

If there is a possibility for us, we will let you know.
The time it goes on learning.

Namasté
Jacqueline Hopstaken (directing the management team and organisation)

I visited Manaltheeram Ayurveda Beach Village in July 2016.

I had the desire to relax from the stress of modern living in a fast-paced city of Dubai. I booked a two week ayurveda package and, as soon as I arrived to the village, I was met with amazing peace and tranquility.

Apart from enjoying the amazing ocean side environment, fresh air and carefully and freshly prepared ayurvedic food, the gusts were also kept under careful daily observations and consultations of Dr. Rajmohan. His expertise in ayurveda was very helpful in reassuring me that I would receive the best possible care while spending time in the village. He was genuinely interested in his patients' well being and strived to get the maximum from all treatments provided.

If I ever get the chance I would certainly go back to Manaltheeram again in the future and undergo treatments under the experienced care of Dr. Rajmohan.

Best Regards,

Andjelka Pavlovic

Marketing Manager, Dubai UAE

Hello Doctor,

Good Day

Myself Suresh s/o Satyam Rongali, am writing this email in appreciation of the advice and treatment received from you for my father's health concerns. We are very grateful to your timely, accurate analysis and treatment on the multiple and complex health concerns for my father, who is suffering from Diabetes and hypertension for the past 25 years and bedridden due to CVA, from beginning of this year.

My father is 75 years old and we have approached multiple doctors for Septic arthritis of his left hip joint, along with his other complications, but couldn't find an alternative to invasive surgical methods. After we approached you for this treatment and started using the prescribed ayurvedic medicines for the last 3 months, his pain levels in the hip joint has substantially decreased and his sugar levels and serum creatinine are well under control. He has regained strength to sit and read newspaper and his books again. We are truly thankful to you for this improvement of his health.

My happiness has no bounds that I could finally convince my family and relatives, who are deep rooted to allopathic system, that Ayurveda truly works in chronic and complicated cases. Am really thankful to you for your critical thought in analysis and care rendered into the treatment and constant ongoing support.

We are very grateful to you and thank you very much.

Thanks and Best Regards,

Suresh

www.ingramcontent.com/pod-product-compliance
Lightning Source LLC
Chambersburg PA
CBHW020852180526
45163CB00007B/2483

APPLICATION GUIDE FOR POWER ENGINEERS

PART 1

EARTHING AND GROUNDING OF ELECTRICAL SYSTEMS

K. RAJAMANI

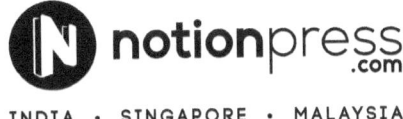

INDIA • SINGAPORE • MALAYSIA

Notion Press

Old No. 38, New No. 6
McNichols Road, Chetpet
Chennai - 600 031

First Published by Notion Press 2018
Copyright © K. Rajamani 2018
All Rights Reserved.

ISBN 978-1-64429-269-3

This book has been published with all efforts taken to make the material error-free after the consent of the author. However, the author and the publisher do not assume and hereby disclaim any liability to any party for any loss, damage, or disruption caused by errors or omissions, whether such errors or omissions result from negligence, accident, or any other cause.

No part of this book may be used, reproduced in any manner whatsoever without written permission from the author, except in the case of brief quotations embodied in critical articles and reviews.